Forward

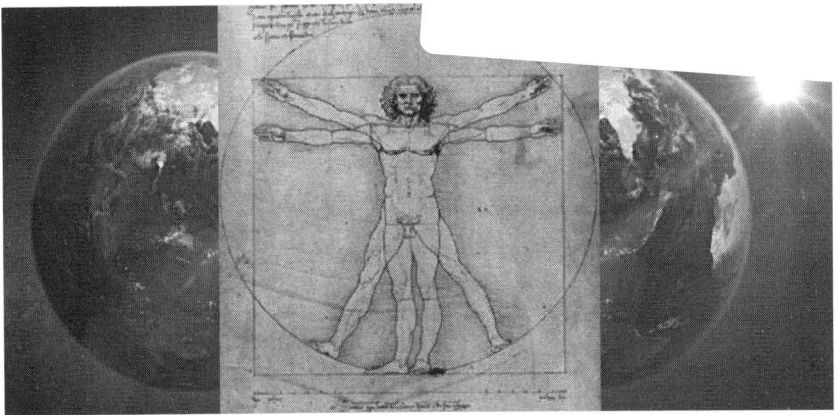

"There may be no individual whose accomplishments were more symbolic of the integration of science and holism than the ultimate Renaissance man, Leonardo da Vinci (1452 - 1519) . Da Vinci's exceptional significance and a reputation was not only due to his brilliant talents in art, but also because he was an exceptional scientist."

" Da Vinci's contributions to our understanding of the universe are that are profound and enduring precisely because of this integration. He realised wholism needed reductionism to advance and reductionism needed wholism to remain relevant. He realised that when you take something out of context to study it more closely or measure it exactly, you risk losing more wisdom than you gain."

Dr. T. Colin Campbell Ph.D "Whole"

This small book attempts to stimulate the reader to regain the faculty of such thinking in a world that has been dominated by reductionism in all fields of study and endeavor, but perhaps most significantly in the field of medicine and healthcare. We are at an critical evolutionary stage in our understanding and practice of medicine and we need to meet this challenge, not with the old paradigm of Newtonian thinking but a new 21st Century Vision, not with Aristotle's "binary" logic but with Buddha's "fuzzy" logic; the former demands something 'is or is not', the latter that something 'is and is not'. This is not the field for the flat-earthers of today!

Contents

Forward		Page 1
Introduction		Page 2
Chapter One	The Body Connection	Pages 3 to 22
Chapter Two	The Food Connection	Pages 23 to 48
Chapter Three	The Breath Connection	Pages 49 to 68
Chapter Four	The Mind Connection	Pages 69 to 76
Chapter Five	The Living Connection	Pages 77 to 88
Chapter Six	The Environment Connection	Pages 89 to 94
References & more resources		Pages 95 to 96
Index		Pages 97 to 99

www.TotalHealthMatters.co.uk

The Connection

There is a widespread idea that Holistic healthcare is something "New Age" and a bit alternative! *Not in the least!* It is the foundation of all great medicine and healthcare since earliest times.

The problem is, that our modern reductionist medicine has driven the best clinical and person centered healthcare out of the normal application and provision of medical care. Great strides have been made in diagnosis, medical & surgical intervention, drug therapy and sophisticated state of the art diagnostic equipment. This is to be applauded as progress, but there has been an erosion of personal caring for the patient who has become "a condition", an "impersonal name" on a computer data bank.
It was Lord Horder who foresaw this process beginning in the 1930's, Dr. Peabody, a renoun physician of the same era, warned against the replacement of care of the patient with increasing technology & efficiency. Today we are discovering the amazing power of our minds in the healing and physiological processes of our bodies.
Holism is slowly returning. This small book aims to stimulate more interest in the amazing connections that relate to our state of health or sickness.
These connections range from physical mechanics of our body through our support of the body with food and breathing and the impact of our mind on our health, to the effect of our close community and family and our whole environment both local and global.

Holism is a tough challenge to aspire to in the field of healthcare but this is truly where the future of medicine and health care lies.

The Body Connection

How's Your Body Knowledge?

Try this simple quiz:

Question 1. Is your body governed by the same Laws of Mechanics as any machine like a clock or motor car?   Yes/No

Question 2. Will a mis-alignment or restriction in your back have a damaging effect on your structure & health?   Yes/No

Question 3. Will a back pain or restriction have an adverse effect on your heart, bladder or stomach?   Yes/No

Question 4. Will most people require some structural work on their back during their lifetime?   Yes/No

Question 5. Can very young children and babies be helped with structural treatment?   Yes/No

If you have ticked every "Yes" then you have a good understanding of the Body Connection.

This chapter will explain how the mechanical state of your body structure can be a major contribution to many health problems besides "Back pain". It will give you the same anatomical and neurological information that every osteopath, physiotherapist or chiropractor is taught.
It will help you understand how a "pain in the neck" or "a pain in the back" may be due to either an internal problem or a structural problem.
It will help you understand these body/health connections better than most medically trained practitioners who have not specialized in structural medicine.
It will give you simple advice as to ways you can help yourself and, just as important, how to decide when to seek professional help.

Good Body Mechanics are the Basis of Good Health.

Look after your body as if it were a Rolls Royce or the finest machine ever built, because it is just that, the most awesome piece of engineering that has taken millions of years to perfect.

The Fundamental Concepts of Body Mechanics

The fundamental concepts of body mechanics are simple:
1. Structure governs function.
2. Function affects structure.
3. The body's structure is a unity.
4. The body heals itself if conditions are right

Structure governs function
We are only recently discovering the almost infinite complexity of the human body; it is perhaps the most amazing "machine" in the Universe and yet mainstream medicine has not recognized this when health is affected by structural problems.

Every machine obeys the same laws of mechanics, a minor misalignment or restriction of a part of a watch or car will have serious effects on its functioning, with parts wearing out, abnormal working or complete cessation. However it appears, that in modern medicine, dominated by drug therapy and reductionism, there is a belief that the human body is unique, in that it will function well regardless of its structural alignment, with perhaps the exception of fractures or dislocations.

Function affects structure
Once we accept the above, it follows that the reverse is also true, that any disturbed function or abnormal activity will have an adverse effect on the structure of the body; from minor local irritation to major pathologies.

The body's structure is a unity
It may not be an exaggeration to say that every cell in our bodies is connected in some way with every other cell, it is easy to understand that, like the old song says, every bone is connected to every other bone. Thus any mechanical problem in one area of the body will produce an effect throughout the entire body. A painful foot will cause one to limp, the awkward, abnormal gait will strain the whole back and even more.

The body heals itself if conditions are right
It has often been said, the physician treats but the body heals. The human body is always working to maintain a state of balanced function. Physical Examinations and Lab Tests are designed to measure those physiologic activities the body keeps constant: Blood pressure, blood sugar, heart rate, etc. all stay within a normal range

The Body Heals Itself if Conditions are Right

Posturally, the body remains balanced in three dimensional space. We can stand on one foot, hold a book in one hand, read, and at the same time bring a cup to our lips without even looking, and without falling over. This is a complex task requiring a constant self-correcting mechanism.

When a patient suffers a laceration, a physician can only assist by cleaning the wound, and bringing the edges together. The healing occurs on its own.

There is within each of us an inherent healing functionality that constantly works to restore homeostasis and body integrity. An integral part of this self-healing process is found in the arterial circulation of our blood. When blood and lymphatics flow freely, tissues can perform their physiologic functions without impedance. With the occurrence of trauma (physical or emotional), the tissues contract, twist, and compress, the fluid flow becomes obstructed. Micro-climates of underperfusion result and are considered to be a significant contributor to the onset of disease. Mechanical adjustment restores freedom in the tissues, normalizes fluid flow and thus inherent physiologic function (healing) follows.

Every cell in our body requires nutrition, oxygenation and protection from foreign viruses or bacteria; the arterial blood carries all these components to every cell where physically possible. Restriction of arterial blood flow, either by physical compression of the blood vessels or by the contraction of smooth muscle tissue from nerve irritation, is perhaps a prime factor in all diseases. It was the recognition of this process that led to the development of osteopathy as a total medical system over a century ago and has since been the basis of all physical therapy positive results.

The Rise of Reductionism and the Fall of Wholism

As our desire to understand the workings of our bodies has grown there has been an increasing focus on smaller and smaller parts of this vital, living thing we call our body. Interestingly it was Lord Horder in his book "Health and a Day" published in 1937, an essential read for every doctor, that he spoke of his fear for the rise of the specialist and the demise of the general practitioner. This combined with increasing mechanization of medicine just making its impact at that time, threatened the future success of medicine.

Getting to Know Your Body

It is quite remarkably that in this information rich world we now live in, just how few people, including doctors, know how our physical structure is intimately connected with our health or disease state. The aim of this book is to try to make this knowledge more available. Why? Only when we know what this connection is can we better help ourselves to better health and aid our recovery from any disease that may afflict us. We will then be able to complement or support any other therapy that we are given.

How can my back pain be connected to my heart problem?

Using the heart as an example, consider the following:

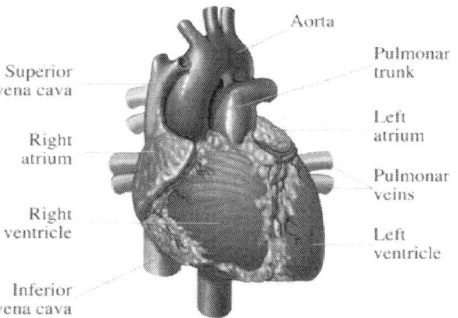

Any nerve root irritation in the neck will alter the nerve supply to the heart, as will problems causing similar irritation in the upper back. These effects can alter the rhythm, beat rate & strength of the heart. Likewise blood supply to and from the heart will be altered with irritated nerve supply to all the blood vessels in the body.

The reverse is also true, that any dysfunction of the heart will cause a change in the tissue corresponding to the nerve supply area of the back. The consequences of this inter-connectedness are that:

1. When there is a tender or painful area in the back we should be aware that it may also be causing a hidden adverse effect on the functioning of any internal organ.
2. That a painful or tender area in the back may be primarily due to a problem in an internal organ and
3. By examinining the back we can aid diagnosis of other health problems and by treating these same areas we can help improve the functioning of the related organs. Once this concept is understood it is easy to see how what seems like just structural treatment, however it is carried out, may have a profound effect on the patient's general health way beyond relieving "the pain in the back".

The Hidden Workings of Your Spine Revealed

The connections understood and used in therapy by every physical therapist. Nerves exiting from each vertebral segment serve specific organs or muscles in the body.

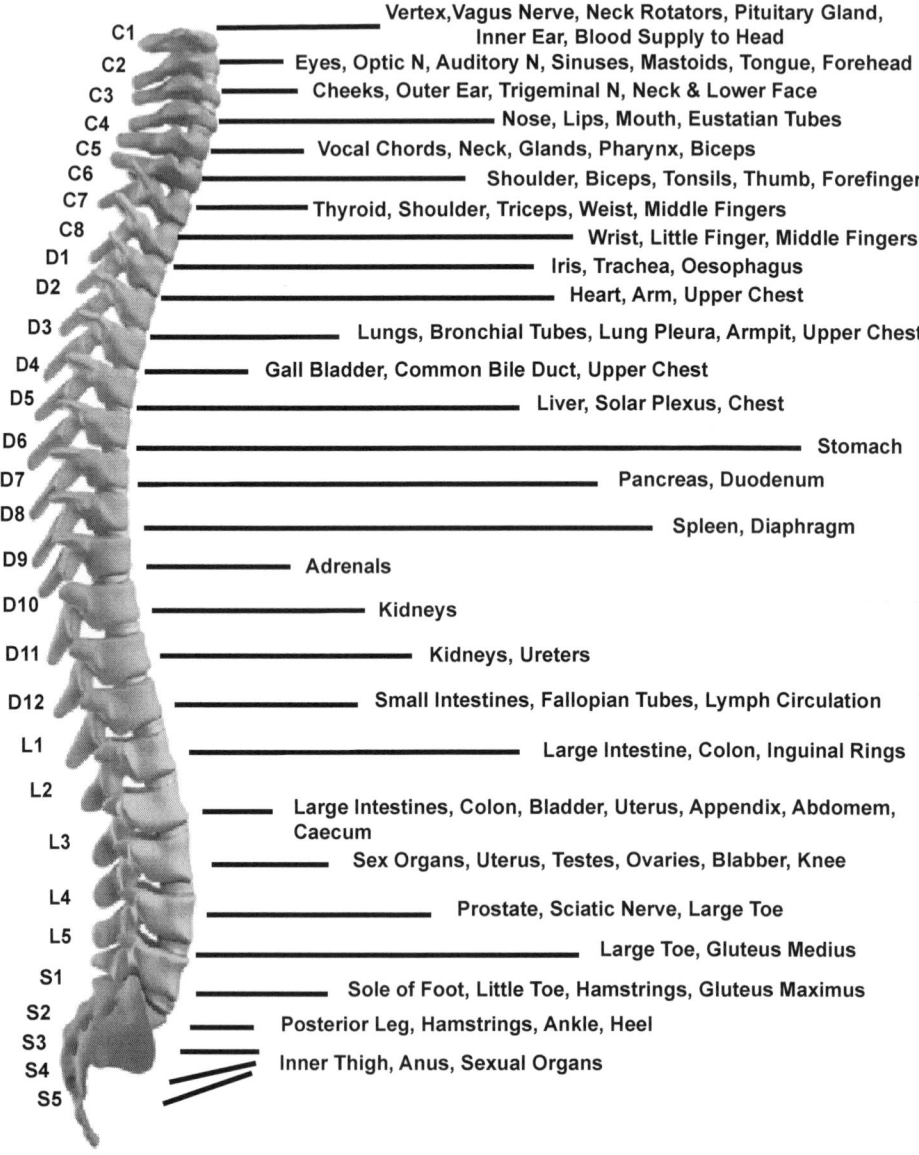

- C1 — Vertex, Vagus Nerve, Neck Rotators, Pituitary Gland, Inner Ear, Blood Supply to Head
- C2 — Eyes, Optic N, Auditory N, Sinuses, Mastoids, Tongue, Forehead
- C3 — Cheeks, Outer Ear, Trigeminal N, Neck & Lower Face
- C4 — Nose, Lips, Mouth, Eustatian Tubes
- C5 — Vocal Chords, Neck, Glands, Pharynx, Biceps
- C6 — Shoulder, Biceps, Tonsils, Thumb, Forefinger
- C7 — Thyroid, Shoulder, Triceps, Weist, Middle Fingers
- C8 — Wrist, Little Finger, Middle Fingers
- D1 — Iris, Trachea, Oesophagus
- D2 — Heart, Arm, Upper Chest
- D3 — Lungs, Bronchial Tubes, Lung Pleura, Armpit, Upper Chest
- D4 — Gall Bladder, Common Bile Duct, Upper Chest
- D5 — Liver, Solar Plexus, Chest
- D6 — Stomach
- D7 — Pancreas, Duodenum
- D8 — Spleen, Diaphragm
- D9 — Adrenals
- D10 — Kidneys
- D11 — Kidneys, Ureters
- D12 — Small Intestines, Fallopian Tubes, Lymph Circulation
- L1 — Large Intestine, Colon, Inguinal Rings
- L2 — Large Intestines, Colon, Bladder, Uterus, Appendix, Abdomem, Caecum
- L3 — Sex Organs, Uterus, Testes, Ovaries, Blabber, Knee
- L4 — Prostate, Sciatic Nerve, Large Toe
- L5 — Large Toe, Gluteus Medius
- S1 — Sole of Foot, Little Toe, Hamstrings, Gluteus Maximus
- S2 — Posterior Leg, Hamstrings, Ankle, Heel
- S3/S4/S5 — Inner Thigh, Anus, Sexual Organs

The Head

The nerve supply to the vertex, forehead, cheeks, mouth and lower face is supplied from the first, second, third and fourth cervical nerves.
Any irritation in these segments of the neck may not only produce pain in the related areas but also disturb the nerve supply of the Vagus nerve that affects the whole digestive system and half of the autonomic system, as well as the nerve supply to the eyes, nose, lips, mouth, sinuses, auditory system and Eustachian tubes.
This segment also supplies nerves to the heart.
Many headaches may arise from these connections as well as certain migraines due to reduced blood flow to the brain.

Neck Pains

Pain can usually be associated with some misalignment or muscle spasm in the cervical vertebrae. Restriction of movement, turning left or right will be noticed as well as local tenderness over the area most affected. Normalisation of the vertebral alignment and movement will usually lead to relief of pain and associated inflammation.
This may be achieved in many ways, using manipulative techniques, release work, or sometimes soft tissue massage.
Note that it is quite common for a neck restriction to be a result of a similar restriction in the lumbar region, that once removed, immediately clears a neck problem. See p18 for a more detailed explanation why this is so.
It is not uncommon for many neck problems to have been caused by stress and the consequent muscle tension in the shoulder area. See the self-help advice on relief of the neck tension.

The Eyes

Nerve supply to the eyes involves the second and third cervical nerves as well as the first thoracic nerve. The latter spinal area is often a problem as it is the junction between the mobile neck and the more fixed first rib. Normalisation of alignment and articulation of this area will benefit the eyesight. This may be achieved in many ways, using soft tissue techniques or other gentle release work. Note neck problems may originate in the lower spine. See also the impact of nutrition and breathing on eyesight in "The Food Connection" and "The Breath Connection" sections.

Facial Pains

Facial pains may involve any of the first four nerves in the neck area. The severe pains associated with trigeminal neuralgia will be specifically linked to the third cervical nerve. Normalisation alignment and articulation of this area should reduced facial pains.

Ear problems

Ear problems will be linked to the nerve supply from the second, third and fourth cervical nerves. The entire ear nose and throat complex may be involved with infections or excessive mucus production in the sinuses that are not freely draining. With regard to "Glue Ear" in children refer to the advice section for specific treatment on page14.

Vocal Chords

Speech and the vocal cords will be linked to the nerve supply from the fifth cervical nerve. Any restrictions in this area will have an adverse affect on voice production. Frequently the vocal chord problems may arise from strain because of dysfunctional breathing, see "The Breath Connection" for more information on this.

Diaphragm

The diaphragm function will be linked to the nerve supply of the fourth, fifth, and sixth cervical nerves as well as the eighth thoracic nerve. The mechanics of breathing are affected by posture, stress and breathing habits. To improve breathing all these aspects may need to be addressed.

Thyroid

Thyroid function will be linked to the nerve supply from the seventh cervical nerve as well as the nutritional status of the body. See "The Food Connection" references for information on diet.

Heart

The heart receives a nerve supply from the second, third cervical nerves & the third and fourth thoracic nerves as well. Although body mechanics have a significant effect on the heart, the most common cause of heart disease is lifestyle; our diet primarily (see "The Food Connection"), our stress and breathing (see "The Breath Connection") as well as inadequate exercise.

Upper Limbs
The upper limbs are served by the fourth to eighth cervical nerves and the first thoracic nerve.

Adrenals
The adrenal is served by the ninth thoracic nerve. Note any stress will increase adrenal activity and stress reduction with breath training may be indicated.

Spleen
The spleen is served by the eighth thoracic nerve.

Kidneys
The kidneys are served by the ninth to twelfth thoracic nerves. Note diet may cause kidney problems, study the Food Connection section for more information and as stress also affects kidney function refer to the Breath Connection for stress management.

Pancreas
The pancreas it is served by the seventh thoracic. Diet has been shown to have a profound effect on pancreatic disease, ideally moving to a whole plant diet with minimal high-fat and oils. See The Food Connection section.

Duodenum
The duodenum is served by the seventh thoracic nerve.

Large Intestine
The large intestine is served by the first and second lumbar nerves. Note dietary factors are prime importance for all conditions affecting the intestine. Study this aspect in the Food Connection. As stress may also have adverse effects in this area related to chronic hidden hyperventilation that causes spasm of smooth muscle wrapped around the intestines. See the Breath Connection for more details on this.

Lungs
Lung function will be linked to the nerve supply from the second to fifth thoracic nerves. The optimal functioning of the lungs is dealt with in detail in the Breath Connection.

Gall Bladder
The gall bladder function will be linked to the supply from the fourth thoracic nerve. Note also the profound impact of diet on gall bladder function in the Food Connection section.

Liver
Liver function is linked to the nerve supply from the sixth to tenth thoracic nerves. Study the impact of diet on the liver function in Food Connection.

Stomach
Stomach function will be linked to the nerve supply from the sixth to the eighth thoracic nerve. Study the impact of diet on this function in the Food Connection section.

Small Intestine
The small intestines nerve supply is from the 12th thoracic nerve. Both diet and stress may have considerable impact on this area, study the Food Connection and the Breath Connection sections.

Heart
The heart receives a nerve supply from the 2nd, 3rd cervical nerves and from the 3rd and 4th thoracic nerves. Most heart diseases today are due to diet and stress. Refer to The Food Connection and The Breath Connection for more details on these connections.

Oesophagus
The oesophagus function will be linked to the nerve supply from the 1st thoracic nerve. Note acid reflux is important and associated with diet & stress, see also The Food Connection & The Breath Connection.

Lymph Circulation
In traditional osteopathic thinking the lymph circulation is controlled by the nerve supply from the 12th thoracic nerve.

Bladder
The bladder's nerve supply involves the 2nd and 3rd lumbar nerves.

Uterus
The uterus is served by the 2nd and 3rd lumbar nerves.

Appendix
The appendix is served by the 2nd lumbar nerve.

Knee
The nerve supply to the knee comes from the 3rd lumbar nerve that is invariably irritated when the pelvis is torsioned, it is one of the main causes of right knee pains. This nerve supply not only causes excess muscle tension around the joint but also it may impair nutrition to the joint due to constriction of the blood vessels serving the area. It is rare for any knee problem not to be connected to a mechanical problem in mid lumbar region.

Abdomen
The main innervation of the abdomen is from the 2nd lumbar nerve.

Prostate
Prostate innervation is derived from the 4th lumbar nerve. Note also that diet has a profound effect on this organ, see The Food Connection for details.

Sciatic Nerve
This large nerve receives branches from the 4th and 5th lumbar nerves and the 1st and 2nd sacral nerves.

Sexual Organs
The 3rd lumbar nerve is closely associated with the sexual organs.

Lower Limbs
The lower limbs are served by all the lumbar and sacral nerves, specific nerves causing problems can be identified by locating the dermatome involved.

Feet
The feet are served by the 4th and 5th lumbar nerves and the 1st and 2nd sacral nerves

Anus
The lower sacral nerves innervate the anus.

Posture

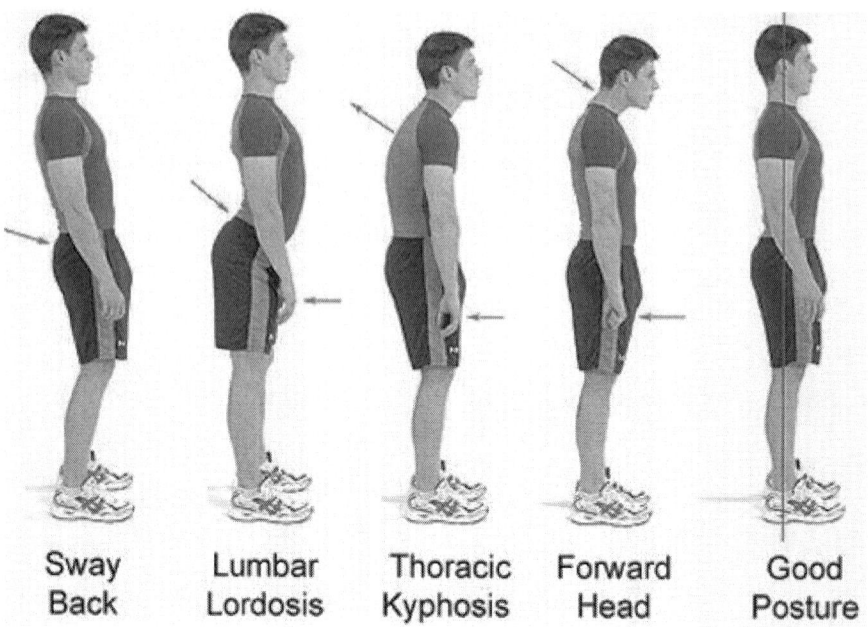

Sway Back | Lumbar Lordosis | Thoracic Kyphosis | Forward Head | Good Posture

The pictures above show the main postural problems that cause further mechanical stresses in the spine and associated health problems.
The most common postural training is The Alexander Technique, but there are many other systems used for training better posture.
The first step is to recognize there is a postural problem and then become more aware of your body 24/7.
Good posture is achieved by lengthening the spine and holding the head level, imagine a helium balloon lifting you from the top of your head level with your ears. Mechanical problems in the spine and pelvis can also be the major cause of poor posture
The impact of poor posture goes beyond mechanical strains to the body but also affects the way we feel; if we feel well and alive we tend to stand tall, whereas if we feel down and depressed we tend to slump. Try these postures and feel the effect on how you feel emotionally.

Children's Structural Problem

A child's structural integrity is just as important as that of the adult, or even more so, as it is a developing structure and minor mechanical problems, if not corrected, can remain a lifelong concern.
Often simple aches and pains complained of by the child are dismissed as "growing pains" or untreated with the expectation that they will "go away" naturally. It is always wise to have persistent musculo-skeletal pains checked out by a trained physical therapist as even children can suffer the kind of back problems adults experience. The parent can make simple checks themselves. With the child standing or lying down note whether there is any marked asymmetry; is one side of the pelvis higher than the other? Is one shoulder higher than the other? Are both feet turned out equally or does one roll out further when lying flat? Can the child side-bend equally easily left and right? Can they turn their head as easily left and right? Any of these restrictions would suggest a mechanical problem needing attention.

Babies

When we consider the potential physical stresses on a baby during their birth it comes as no surprise that many babies often suffer from symptoms due to mechanical strains at birth that may include; colic, poor ability to feed, poor disturbed sleep, general irritability and other signs of general discomfort. These problems can be helped with Cranio-Sacral therapy. Perhaps the most common reason for such problems is due to the compression of the head onto the atlas while passing through the birth canal, especially if the birth was particularly long and difficult or at the other extreme, easy and very fast for the mother. The passage through the birth canal should be a beneficial process that gently compresses and releases the cranial structures, removing any strain patterns developed while in the womb. Thus babies delivered by Cesarian section miss out on this natural de-stressing process and may therefore also need some attention soon after birth. Cranio-Sacral Treatment is very gentle and effective, usually giving noticeable benefit within days. Parents can be taught how to do some work to aid this process.

Glue Ear

This common childhood problem, blocking of the Eustation tubes with mucus is frequently treated by surgical implanting grommets in the ear. It responds well to physical treatment done by the parent with guidance from their osteopath.

Always try eliminating dairy produce as a first step as many children produce excess mucus when fed dairy produce. See The Food Connection for more information about the health hazards of milk and that it is not the best source of calcium or protein for children.

View Dr. Tony Matthew's video showing how this well proven procedure for glue ear is done in practice. <https://vimeo.com/12749323>

Orthodontics

It comes as a surprise to most people that many orthodontic problems can be avoided or helped with structural therapy and breath training. The development of the head structures in a child influences the development of the body and vice versa.

By normalising the structure with physical therapy, often cranio-sacral therapy, and by teaching the child to breathe normally most orthodontic problems of crooked teeth can be avoided.

The connection with breathing and orthodontic problems can be easily demonstrated on yourself as follows. Firstly you must know that a very small force of just a few grams can move a tooth if applied 24/7; this is how orthodontic braces work. Now just breathe normally through your mouth and note where your tongue is placed. Unless you are very unusual it will be lying on your lower teeth. Now breathe normally through your nose and note where your tongue is again. You will feel it pressing upwards on the roof of your mouth, where it is applying about 30 grams pressure 24/7 if you normally breathe through your nose. In the developing child this constant gentle pressure ensures normal structural development of your child's teeth and entire facial bone alignment; producing normal well-formed facial features. This is an interesting cross-over of the Breath and Body connections.

To learn more about this relationship visit an excellent video lecture by Dr. John Flutter at <https://youtu.be/tVjMgVClyPA> and see more in The Breath Connection section.

Babies and how you can help

A cranio-sacral therapy is the most effective approach for any birth trauma but the parent could try two simple procedures with total safety and often remarkable success.
Method One: Whilst the baby is lying down and asleep or resting just place your hand under its head to cradle and support it, with the pads of your fingers gently touching the base of the skull. Hold this position for a minute or two, then release. If done successfully you will notice your baby stretch & relax almost immediately. You are effectively reducing the compression strain mentioned above. It may take a few sessions over a few days to release all the strain pattern.

Method Two: This requires a conceptual leap for many people but if you can overcome your intellectual barriers it can be a great help releasing complex strain patterns in the membranes of the baby's brain and is safe. When your baby is asleep or lying still, place your hands a little distance from either side of the baby's head (about half an inch or so) and make yourself relaxed and focussed on trying to feel any sensations that may come from the baby's head. If you begin to feel a heat release you are almost certainly causing a release of physical tensions in the head and your child will respond positively to this. If you don't feel any sensations it may simply mean that there are no significant stress patterns in the baby's head. If you still feel your baby needs help in this way try to find a therapist who is trained in cranio-sacral therapy.

Young Children

Young children respond quickly and well to structural treatment as their mechanical problems are usually less well established than an adult's and often the adult problem in the spine is also a reponse to stress and poor body posture. If the child complains of pains worse for activity but easier for rest and there are tender areas along the spine that match the pains complained of, then it is likely there are structural problems needing attention. This would apply to many pains occuring in the knees or feet as well as the back.

Boosting your child's immune sysyem

There is a simple way of boosting your child's immune response to any infection by mobilizing their immune system physically. The immune system is carried around the body by the lymph circulation and the main source of the lymphatic fluid is held in the lymph gland in the upper chest.
For babies, use just two fingers placed in the centre of the upper chest and gently depress and release over this area with the minimum pressure to cause a pumping action on the lymph gland every few seconds for a minute. Repeat every hour or so during the day. Research has shown this lymph pump can double the circulation of our immune system.
With older children the same procedure applies but the pumping may be done with the whole hand, once again only sufficient pressure to gently move the chest to create the pumping effect. If in doubt consult a physical therapist for a practical demonstration. Needless to say diet and breathing will impact on the child's immune capacity as well.

Earache relief

Any earache usually indicates congestion and infection in the inner ear. Relief may be given by improving the circulation in this area as follows. With the person lying down or sitting, hold both ears and pull away from the head as gently as possible, almost just "thinking of pulling". This is a technique that proves the concept that "less is more", as any heavy pulling will aggravate the problem but very gentle release will ease the pain and improve local circulation. Should the pain persist and worsen consult your doctor to confirm there is no more serious problem causing the pain.

Is your knee problem really a knee problem?

The knee is primarily a simple hinge joint that has the capacity to rotate a few degrees when standing upright in order to provide support with minimum muscle avtivity. Most knee problems that have not been preceded by physical trauma & injury are due to stresses arising from the misalignment of the body structures. Just like the hinges on a door, that function well so long as they have been fitted correctly, square with the door post, so it is with the knee joint. If the pelvis is tilted due to a torsion of the sacroiliac joint the knees will not be able to hinge freely without twisting and straining the joint.

Besides this the nerve supply to the knee will have been irritated from the third lumbar region causing muscle imbalance around the joint as well as impaired blood supply to the tissues. If this were all it would explain most pains in the knees but in addition the load bearing on the knees is totally changed when the pelvis is tilted. This may cause a strain to the inner part of the right knee, affecting ligament and cartilage there and also excessive weight bearing on the left knee that is almost permanently fully extended in an attempt to bring the pelvis back to level.
Correction of the pelvis and lumbar areas will invariably remove the pain and stress on the knees. This is the standard work of a physical therapist such as osteopath or chiropractor.

Is your neck problem really a low back problem?

It is often difficult for people to understand that the site of a pain is not always the area responsible for the pain.
The spine operates as a unified structure, rather like a suspension bridge, if one end of the bridge twists due to collapse of one foundation this twist will be conveyed to the opposite side instantly.
Thus if there is a problem in the low back showing as a tilt on the pelvis, the lumbar vertebrae will side-bend to the opposite side to try to compensate for the tilt and bring the body upright again. This shift in the lumbar vertebrae will produce a similar shift in the opposite end of this "suspension bridge" and cause the neck vertebae to rotate and side-bend in a similar way.
There may be little or no pain from the low back but the neck restriction may be causing considerable pain that will also affect the whole upper limb function as well.
Correction of the pelvis and low back will usually correct the painful neck problem with little or no direct treatment of that area. Likewise if treatment is only directed to the neck, the problem may well return again and again while ever the low back is out of alignment.
It may also be true that in some instances the low back, pelvis or hip pain may originate from mechanical strains in the upper back or neck as for instance after a whiplash injury. This simply emphasises the need to treat the entire spine rather than any single segment.

A Story about Pain Killers & The Red Flashing Light

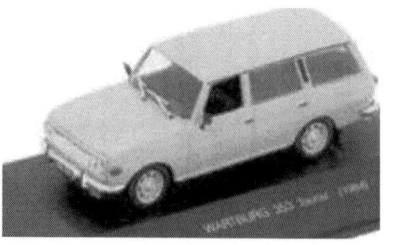

The author of this book once owned a secondhand East German car called a Wartburg when a student. It had an unfortunate habit of showing a red flashing light on the dashboard that was very distracting when driving at night. Tired of this irritation he solved the problem by covering the offending light with a sticking plaster; comfortable night driving was thus resumed.

Only when the car was taken in for its MOT and service was it discovered that there was very little oil in the engine and had he continued to drive a few more miles the engine would have been seriously damaged.

When people hear this true story they comment how stupid can you get! Didn't he realize the red flashing light was the indicator that there was a oil level problem that needed urgent attention? His reply was usually that he was only doing what most people do, often with good professional advice, when they have a pain; they cover the pain with a pain killer.

They disregard the fact that the pain is the body's flashing red light indicating something needs urgent attention. Admitted there may be exceptions, as for instance when sleep is disturbed by the pain or when there is chronic pain that has a untreatable pathological origin, but the casual use of pain killers is as unreasonable as the sticking plaster on the oil warning light.

How do I know I need physical therapy?

Let's start with a broad generalization, most of us will benefit from an annual physical MOT to ensure our mechanics are in good order, we are all used to having our car checked this way why not our body structure that is infinitely more complex?

Although it is actually quite difficult to diagnose oneself with regard to body mechanics, here are a few simple tips you may try:

Standing in front of a mirror check "Are your shoulders absolutely level?"
Laying on your back on the floor "Do your legs swing to one side?" and
" Does your right foot roll outwards more than your left foot?"
Is it more difficult to turn your head to the left or to the right?
Is it more difficult to side-bend to the left or to the right when standing ?
A "Yes" to any of these questions suggests you have some mechanical

restrictions that may be adversely affecting your health.
If you have any pain in joints or muscles that is worse for movement but eases with rest this would be a reasonable indicator that you would need some physical therapy.
There is a more difficult area for consideration and that is where you have a headache, migraine, internal pains, chest pains and a whole range of other health problems that may be relatively benign and would benefit from good physical treatment, perhaps combined with other lifestyle changes, or might be indicators of more serious pathologies that need medical investigation and additional tests.
Here it is wise to first eliminate the possiblity of the more serious health problem by consulting your doctor and then discussing whether some physical therapy would complement any medical treatment being prescribed. Remember that even the more serious health problems will always have an impact on the structure and mechanics in some way, perhaps just a slight muscular pain, an inflammatory reaction in the back causing tension, increased muscle tension disturbing the structural integrity or just impaired mobility. Professional, judicious help with these mechanical problems will support and aid any other treatment being received.

Can I exercise my mechanical problems away?

This is a very contentious area for discussion but certain points can be made to help provide an answer.
First, if the back is in good mechanical alignment there is little argument that regular careful exercise will help keep it in good order, this might be simply a little brisk walking, housework, Pilates, Tai Chi, Yoga, stretching exercises and any physical recreation or sport that does not put undue strain on the back or involve physical injury.
If however there are significant mechanical problems in the back, restrictions, misalignments, areas of excessive muscle tension, painful joints or muscles, or anything that makes normal mobility difficult the answer is probably: "Do not try to exercise the problem away". If you presented your garage with your car and a misalignment of the wheels you would not be impressed if told to drive it repeatedly around a circuit to fix the problem! Like most complex problems there are the exceptions to any rule and this is true here. Carefully selected exercises may well maintain or improve joint function as part of an overall structural treatment.

How do you choose a physical therapist?

> ?Tai Chi ? Sports Massage?Yoga?Bowen Technique?Osteopathy?Physiotherapy?Alexander Technique?Chiropractic?Cranio-Sacral Therapy?Exercise therapy?

This is much more difficult to answer than trying to find a doctor or dentist although there are similar questions to ask. The reason for this difficulty is also an indication of the value of this question. As a broad generalisation doctors and dentists are a relatively homogeneous group, well defined by their professional bodies and all having received very similar education & training. Physical therapy, on the other hand, embraces a vast variety of approaches and methods all of which may be appropriate for certain specific conditions and patients some of the time but not for all patients all the time. One of the gentlest physical therapies is cranio-sacral therapy that works on the minute movements of the cranial structures and related flow of cerebro-spinal fluid throughout the body, soft tissue massage may be light to heavy therapy, osteopathy and chiropractic involve mechanical adjustment of structures using a wide variety of techniques and physiotherapy is perhaps the most widely known system of physical therapy that besides physical treatment, engages the patient in exercise routines as well. The Alexander Technique teaches improved posture and body use. Other approaches that improve or maintain body mechanics include Yoga, Tai Chi and Pilates. Perhaps the best way of choosing a therapy or therapy is by recommendation by your doctor or friend who has experienced a similar problem to you and had benefit from that approach.

There is no single unique way to treat a back and each therapy brings a different approach to this highly complex biological machine. You need to discover for yourself what suits you personally by experiencing some of the many approaches mentioned above. Some therapists may be happy to give you a free consultation to discuss your specific health problem and to explain what & how they might help you.

The Demise of Physical Therapy (Osteopathy in Particular)

The author trained as an osteopath in 1981 at the European School of Osteopathy in Maidstone, Kent. The course was excelent as students were trained by a wide spectrum of experienced practitioners from the most traditional to the most modern. However over the past 25 years osteopathy has suffered a serious dilution of its original potential and standing despite the Statutory Regulation that should have opened the doors to full incorporation into our NHS. To highlight this professional demise it may be of interest to recall the words of Andrew Taylor Still, the founder of osteopathy:

"It should be known where osteopathy stands and what it stands for. A political party has a platform that all may know its position in regard to matters of public importance, what it stands for and what principles it advocates. The osteopath should make his position just as clear to the public. He should let the public know, in his platform, what he advocates in his campaign against disease. Our position can be tersely stated in the following planks:
1. We believe in sanitation and hygiene.**(Still incorporated)**

2. We are opposed to the use of drugs as remedial agencies. **(No longer incorporated)**

3. We are opposed to vaccination. **(No longer incorporated)**

4. We are opposed to the use of serums in the treatment of disease. Nature furnishes its own serum if we know how to deliver them. **(No longer incorporated)**

5. We realize that many cases require surgical treatment and therefore advocate it as a last resort. We believe many surgical operations are unnecessarily performed and that many operations can be avoided by osteopathic treatment. **(Still incorporated)**

6. The osteopath does not depend on electricity, X--radiance, hydrotherapy or other adjuncts, but relies on osteopathic measures in the treatment of disease. **(No longer incorporated)**

7. We have a friendly feeling for other non--drug, natural methods of healing, but we do not in-corporate any other methods into our system. We are all opposed to drugs; in that respect at least, all natural, un-harmful methods occupy the same ground. The fundamental principles of osteopathy are different from those of any other system and the cause of disease is considered from one standpoint, viz.: disease is the result of anatomical abnormalities followed by physiological discord.To cure disease the abnormal parts must be adjusted to the normal; therefore other methods that are entirely different in principle have no place in the osteopathic system. **(No longer incorporated)**

8. Osteopathy is an independent system and can be applied to all conditions of disease, including purely surgical cases, and in these cases surgery is but a branch of osteopathy. **(No longer incorporated)**

9. We believe that our therapeutic house is just large enough for osteopathy and that when other methods are brought in just that much osteopathy must move out." **(No longer incorporated)**
From "Osteopathy Research and Practice? by A Taylor Still 1910

There may be good reason why osteopathy has rejected some of the old concepts but in truth the profession has been diminished beyond recognition and it is a sad reflection on the medical establishment that NHS osteopathy is not yet available.

The Food Connection

Visit <www.TheFoodConnection.org.uk> to access this map below where you may click on any condition to learn more from leading doctors, watch their video talks or access the latest research.

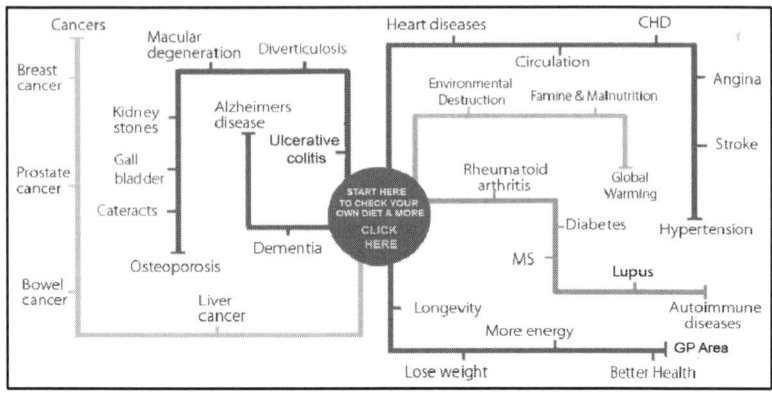

The question you need to ask yourself is:

"Would it make good sense to change ones lifestyle and eating habits if all, or most of the following benefits were likely to ensue?"

To live a longer, healthy, active life.	Avoid surgery in many instances
Look and feel younger.	Preserve your eyesight in your later years
To have more energy.	
Lose weight, if you're overweight.	Prevent and treat diabetes
Lower your blood cholesterol.	Vastly decrease the need for pharmaceutical drugs
Prevent or reverse heart disease.	
Lower your risk of prostate, breast or other cancers	To keep your bones strong
	Avoid a stroke Avoid impotence
Lower your blood pressure	Prevent kidney stones
Reduce the risk of dementia	Beat arthritis, and much more.....

The science is clear. The results are unmistakable.
Change your diet and dramatically reduce your risk of cancer, heart disease, diabetes, obesity and all the above.

The choice is literally in your hands - your knife and fork!

You are what you eat!

Why not give yourself all the background & hard facts, then you'll be able to make an informed decision as to whether it is worth making a progressive change to your eating habits over the next few weeks or years? Most of us don't like making changes in our diet that we may have followed for decades. There is a certain amount of "addiction" to the foods we eat regularly and we need to recognize this problem when it comes to trying to make any changes. Read "The Pleasure Trap" by Douglas L Lisle.

This is not about a new radical diet that everyone should follow, like the hundreds of other diets that have been fashionable from time to time; *it is about giving you the best research information about how our food intake relates to our health and wellbeing or our sickness & disease.* There are still many questions to be answered on this subject but *the information given here is based on the most comprehensive experimentation & research ever done in the field of nutrition.*

Does it really matter what I eat?

This depends on what your personal priorities are. You may decide that you will not change any of your eating habits whatever the long term health consequences may be. You know what you like and that is what you will continue eating; *in which case this is not for you!*
On the other hand you may want to know how you could deal with some of the health problems you may already have or how to try to avoid other serious health problems that you have seen ruin to the lives of relatives or friends you know, even some young people.
Are most illnesses just a matter of bad luck & genes or do we really have a significant role to play in our own health and lives? The answer is a very positive "**Yes**, *we can determine our health and life quality to a remarkable extent if only we know how & are willing to act on that knowledge*" However there is no 100% certainty that the worst diet will lead to a serious disease & early death or that the best diet will protect everyone. It's all about the degree of risk.

Ref.A1

Start by checking your own diet

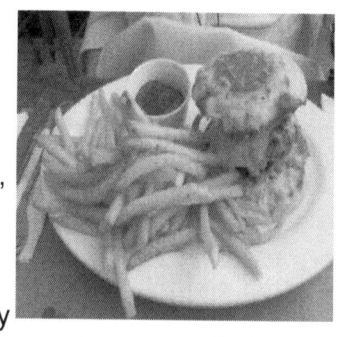

There are many ways of checking people's diet depending on what are considered the key factors in the diet; we could try to assess the detailed nutritional content down to every vitamin, mineral and amino acid or just the variety of diet or any other analysis based on a specific diet being promoted. The simple approach used here is called the "4LeafSurvey" and was developed by eCornell University as a quick guide to where a person is on a scale from - 40 to + 40 that roughly corresponds to the balance between two extreme diets. At one end there is what might be called the "Affluent American Diet", based on plenty of meat, dairy, refined foods, convenience foods, snacks, fizzy drinks, rich creamy desserts and large portions of all of these, and at the other end there is a diet, that a large proportion of the world's population eat, that is based on vegetables, fruit, pulses, grains, legumes, nuts, seeds, tubers, all unrefined and in plenty. As a rough guide you will find the usual UK "Meat and Two Veg." diet will sit somewhere in the middle with a score of between - 10 and + 10 depending on what else is eaten.

Do not regard this survey as a competetive test but more as a measuring tool to guide you to healthier eating, according to the concepts and research findings outlined in this book.

The 4LeafSurvey

The best way of completing this survey would be on line, by logging onto the following site: <http://www.ecornell.com/4Leaf-Survey/> where you will be given instructions and learn your score automatically once you have completed the survey.

Alternatively you may use the questionnaire on the next page and calculate your own score manually. This may not be as accurate but will suffice for a useful guide as you make changes in your diet.

Either way, once you have your 4LeafSurvey Score you will then be able to see where you are on the Schematic Health Risk Graph on page 27.

Note that this is only a broad guide and that it may well be possible that a person with the worst score from an affluent excessive diet who drinks too much alcohol and smokes may not suffer any serious illness and live a long life, just as a person who lives an exemplary life might still suffer a serious disease.

The 4LeafSurvey *(Based on the eCornell University Internet Site)*

The 4Leaf Survey was designed to help people everywhere to make the shift to maximizing the %age of their calories from whole, plant-based foods. For each statement, choose the word or phrase that best characterizes how you actually behave.
Note: A serving = about ¼ plate, an apple, half cup berries, etc..

1. Fresh fruit. On average **how many daily servings** of whole fresh fruit do you eat? (Fruit juice doesn't count, it is not whole fruit)

	None	1-2	3-5	6+
Score	-4	0	+4	+6

2. Whole vegetables. On average, **how many daily servings** of whole vegetables do you eat?

	None	1-2	3-5	6+
Score	-4	0	+4	+6

3. Whole grains (brown rice, oats etc.), legumes (peas/beans/pulses), potatoes or other starches. On average, **how many daily servings** of these foods do you eat?

	None	1-2	3-5	6+
Score	-4	+2	+4	+6

4. Omega-3's. Are you getting all you need from whole plant food sources like flaxseeds, walnuts, hemp & chia seeds?

	No	Not sure	Maybe	Yes
Score	-1	0	+1	+2

5. Dairy foods. How many days per week do you eat dairy foods like cheese, yogurt and ice cream? (Soya does not count)

	None	1-2	3-5	6+
Score	+4	+2	-2	-4

6. Eggs. How many days per week do you either eat eggs or add as an ingredient when cooking?

	None	1-2	3-5	6+
Score	+4	+2	-2	-4

7. Cow's milk or cream. How many days per week do you drink them or add them to your food, like cereals, coffee etc.?

	None	1-2	3-5	6+
Score	+4	+2	-2	-4

8. Added sugar. Are you really serious about eliminating added sugar at home and in food products that you buy?

	Yes, really	Fairly	Not very	No
Score	+2	+1	-2	-3

9. White refined flour. (Bread, pasta, cakes, biscuits, etc.) How would you describe your consumption of these foods?

	Zero	Light	Medium	Heavy
Score	+2	-1	-2	-3

10. Sweet and/or salty Processed Snacks. How would you best describe your consumption of these unhealthy foods?

	Minimal	Light	Medium	Heavy
Score	+2	-1	-2	-3

11. Meat, poultry and fish. How many of your meals per week include any animal flesh? (Beef, pork, lamb, chicken, turkey or fish)

	0-1	2-5	6-11	12+
Score	+2	-2	-4	-6

12. Vegetable oil. How many of your meals per week include vegetable oil, like olive or canole? (All oil is 100% fat, not whole plant)

	0-1	2-5	6-11	12+
Score	+1	0	-1	-2

Your total score____
(Now check this against the health risk chart on page 26 & start to change your diet to move towards a better, health promoting and disease protective diet.)

What is Your Health Risk with Your Present Diet?

The potential risk of diseases such as Alzheimer's Disease, Autoimmune diseases, Angina, Arthritis, Bowel Cancer, Breast Cancer, CHD, Diabetes, Hypertension, Liver Cancer, Lupus, MS, Osteoporosis, Prostate Cancer, Rheumatoid Arthritis, Stroke, and many more is closely linked to our diet.

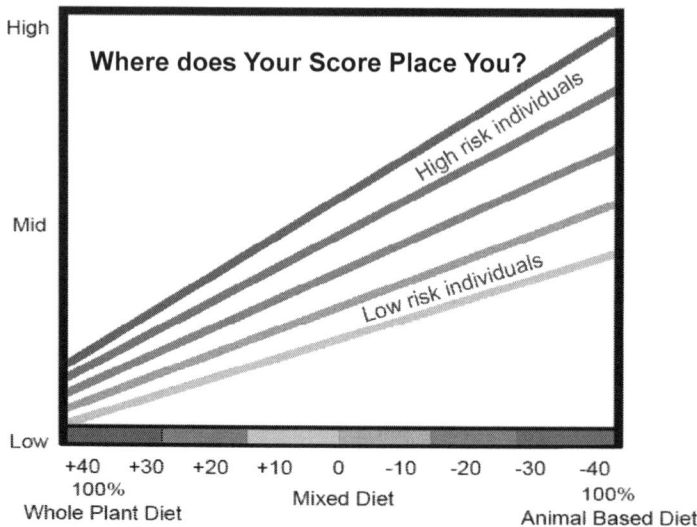

As our diet changes from a dominant animal food based diet towards a whole plant diet the 4LeafSurvey Score goes from -40 towards +40 & general health & wellbeing usually improve along with the reducing risk of slowly developing the serious long term illnesses noted above.

Note: the above schematic diagram gives a very simplified risk assessment of various mixed diets. Remember that even a 100% WPBD does not guarantee freedom from any health risk. A very small % age is due to our genetic make-up (about 2%), environmental factors etc. Likewise a 100% ABFD does not guarantee you will suffer a major modern disease, just as some people have been able to live an active life to 95 years of age smoking 40 cigarettes a day and heavy drinking, but they are the exception! You don't have to make a radical change in your diet unless your health is seriously troubling you, just take small steps in the right direction on a day to day basis. Every move to the left, towards a whole plant diet, can only be a shift towards better health and a longer, active life.

Better Health & A Long Active Life

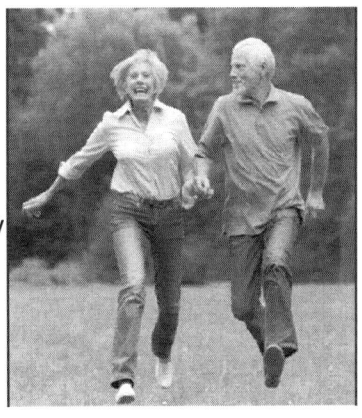

If you have ever wondered what are the key factors that determine our health and longevity and would like some practical, reliable, information on this subject then read on. It is unfortunate that modern medicine has been primarily concerned with disease, illness and pathology for the past century and has not given the public much advice on health promotion. The main reason for this omission, is that doctors are not trained as health practioners; they receive very little training in *the fundamentals of health promotion: the need for good body mechanics, for good nutrition, for adequate exercise, good breathing, good relaxation, a healthy environment and a supportive community.*
Because of this disease model of medical practice, the system is overloaded with a sick population that is creating increasingly impossible demands on finance and resources.
We also have trained an entire generation of the public to rely on their doctor to keep them well and have lost the sense of self-responsibility for their own health or are just unwilling to do anything to help themselves.
There is today a prevalent view that "It's pointless worrying about our own health and quality of life or longevity, just carry on & enjoy yourself as we all have to die of something don't we?" The truth is we can have a profound effect on our health and longevity and we can usually choose either a long healthy, active life or a chronically sick existence for many years maintained with increasing medical & surgical interventions.

If we follow the American lifestyle over the next few years we can expect the same outcomes; according to good medical authority we may be seeing parents routinely outliving their children for the first time in our history. It is now commonplace in America for young people to be suffering strokes or heart attacks and other chronic degenerative diseases that were usually the diseases of middle or old age in the past. The major reason for this catastrophic decline in health and increased premature death appears to be largely due to diet, lack of exercise & an unhealthy lifestyle with increasing medical interventions with drugs and surgery. The brief notes that follow explain some of the research that has led to these conclusions.

Ref.A2

Allergies

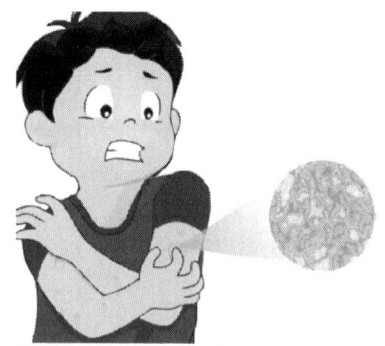

Allergies range over a vast field of possible causes and any detailed study would be impossible in this short book. If we just look at food allergies we can narrow the problem down as there appear to be a relatively small number of common foods that are the most common cause of this problem. They include: Cow's milk (the most common food allergen), Eggs, Shellfish & Peanuts (more common), Fish, Tree nuts, Fruits (common) & Wheat & Soya (less common).

The earliest medical research into this subject was by Dr. Richard Mackarness in 1980 with his ground-breaking book that first put food allergy onto the medical agenda, entitled "Not All In the Mind - How Unsuspected Food Allergy Can Affect Your Body and Your Mind" Since then, this has become a new medical "industry" with numerous clinics & practitioners offering a wide variety of testing systems. Perhaps the first step to take if an allergic problem is suspected is to eliminate all dairy food for a week or so and see whether symptoms go. This will help a large proportion of sufferers. Cow's milk although promoted for many years as the best source of nutrition, is in fact more often the source of many health problems in all age groups.

Alzheimer's Disease & Dementia

Progressive impairment of brain activity whether memory loss or impaired ability to think clearly is not due to a single factor. There are many links between minor strokes, cardio-vascular diseases, hypertension, high blood cholesterol, inadequate physical and mental activity, genetics, low levels of antioxidants in the blood, and high levels of free radicals.

Of all these factors there is a common thread running through most of them and that involves the diet. A whole plant diet offers increased protection against minor strokes, cardio-vascular diseases, hypertension, high blood cholesterol, poor levels of antioxidants, and reduces the levels of free radicals. Whereas a predominantly animal based diet does just the opposite. All research of groups eating a high plant based diet show lower rates of Alzheimer disease, this surely is a useful guide to improved long term health?

Ref.A2

Angina

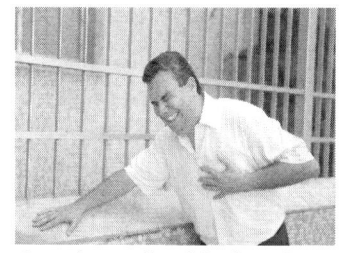

Angina is a condition that produces debilitating chest pain due to restricted blood flow to the arteries of the heart. This reduced blood flow is in part due to a build up of fatty deposits within the walls of the cardiac arteries and may also involve the consequent constriction of arterial blood vessels throughout the body due to lowered carbon dioxide levels arising from hyperventilation. The damage and narrowing of the blood vessels is explained in the Heart Disease section & information on the effect of hyperventilation on circulation & angina can be seen in the section "The Breath Connection". Ref.A3

Arthritis

Osteoarthritis is found to be associated with diet, physical exercise & body mechanics. If we eliminate the excessive abnormal stresses on our joints due to mechanical misalignments and any specific over use of joints due to repetitive work activity we are left with the possibility that most osteoarthritis is associated with quality of bone. The bone quality appears to be related to our diet and normal nutrition from blood supply to the joints affected. Research indicates that a high Bone Mass Density increases the risk of osteoarthritis and that a high animal food based diet increases the risk of fractures due to osteoporosis and excessive calcium excretion.
See also Osteoporosis and Rheumatoid Arthritis. Ref. A4

Auto-immune Diseases

Autoimmune diseases all have common features that include:
A dysfunctional body immune system that attacks itself, they are more common in higher latitudes where there is less sunshine and consequently lower levels of Vitamin D, they tend to associated with other autoimmune conditions in the same people, all those diseases that have been studied for a nutritional connection show an association with consumption of animal protein, especially cow's milk, and there is evidence that a virus may trigger the disease. At this time there is no clear evidence from research that the above factors raise the risk of autoimmune diseases but there is a simple idea that some might agree with; if by changing our dietary habits and by carefully increasing our time in the sun there may be

Auto-immune Diseases continued
a beneficial effect of protecting us from these diseases, why not, as there are no risks from doing so?

For individuals already afflicted with an autoimmune disease a change of diet could be tried for a month or so and they could then ascertain for themselves whether or not they experienced any health improvement or reduction in symptoms. Nothing would be lost.

Ref.A5

Bowel Cancer
There is a wide variation of colorectal or large bowel cancer between countries, deaths from this cause are roughly three times greater in developed countries than under-developed countries. From many studies, meat has been found to be the prime factor linked to these wide variations.

The chart below shows incidence of female colon cancer and dietary meat consumption by country:

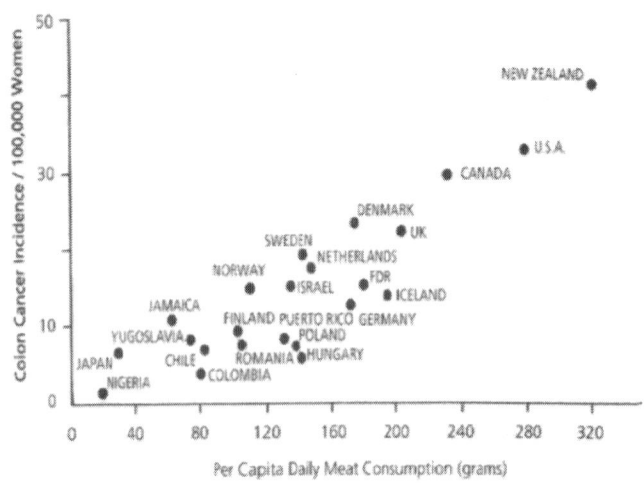

From "The China Study" by T. Colin Campbell & Thomas M. Campbell p.85

The debate still continues as to what are the key factors that protect us from this cancer; is it fibre, fruit, vegetables, carbohydrates, calcium, physical exercise or what? A whole plant diet provides all these nutrients automatically. What has been shown in many studies is wherever dietary fibre is high colon cancer is lower, exactly what it is in the fibre that reduces this risk

Bowel Cancer continued

is not yet known, but it would seem to make good sense for anyone at risk to increase their dietary fibre. That means more fruit, vegetables, legumes, beans etc.

Ref.B1

Breast Cancer

There are a number of generally accepted risk factors connected with breast cancer that include the following:
1. Early age of first menstruation.
2. Late menopause.
3. High blood cholesterol.
4. High levels of female hormones.
5. The ratio of animal-based food to whole plant-based food in diet.

The evidence gathered over the last two decades shows that factor 5 influences all the other factors and that the incidence of breast cancer appears to be linked to the level of animal-based food in the diet. See chart below:

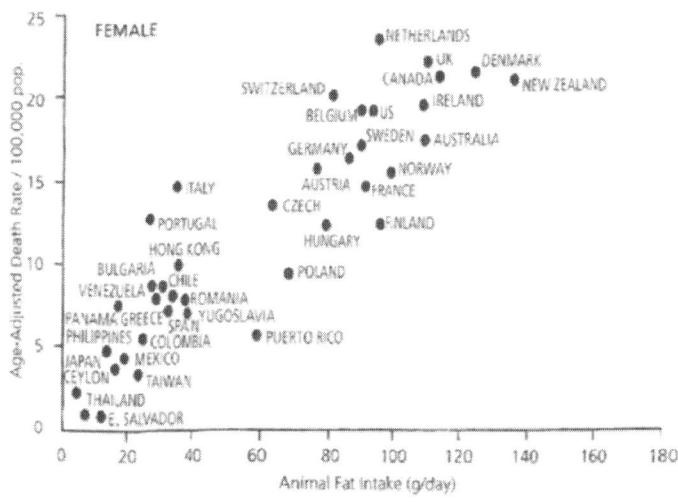

CHART 4.8: ANIMAL FAT INTAKE AND BREAST CANCER

From "The China Study" by T.Colin Campbell & Thomas M. Campbell p.85

Ref B2

Circulation

Normal healthy circulation depends upon healthy blood vessels, normal blood pressure, a healthy heart and normal breathing. Factors influencing the heart, blood vessels and blood pressure are covered in the individual topics. More information showing the connection between circulation & breathing can be found in "The Breath Connection" section.

Coronary Heart Disease

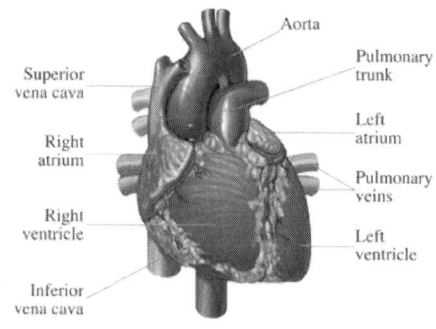

The most common cause of death in the West is a heart attack; in America over 40% of deaths are caused by a heart attack, *more than any other disease or injury including cancer.* Every 24-hour some 3000 Americans will have a heart attack, roughly the same number that died in the September 11th 2001 terrorist attack.

Heart disease used to be a condition of old age, today it is increasingly found among young people and even children. A study of 300 male soldiers in their 20's who had died in action had their hearts examined and it was found that 77% had evidence of gross heart disease.

What is heart disease?

Most heart disease is associated with a narrowing of arteries supplying blood to the heart due to the slow deposition of fatty plaque. At some point this hidden problem goes critical and forms a blockage of a vital artery causing the heart attack. We now know what are the main causes of a heart attack. Risk factors include the following:

1. **High cholesterol level in the blood. (Statins are *not* the answer).**
2. **Stress.**
3. **High blood pressure.**
4. **Smoking.**
5. **Lack of physical exercise.**
6. **Overweight or obesity.**

Of all these factors the most reliable predictor of heart disease is elevated cholesterol levels in the blood. Elevated blood cholesterol is linked to consumption of animal based fats. (Cholesterol nil in plant based foods but high in animal based foods)

Smoking and high blood pressure are also related to stress in people's lives and as stress has a profound effect on our health this should always be addressed and managed. Read "The Breath Connection" section to discover a proven way of combating the ill effects of stress through Breath Training.

Thousands of scientific papers been published concerning the dietary impact on heart disease and perhaps the major relationship that is almost universally agreed as a predictor of heart disease is the cholesterol levels in the body. The following graph shows the link from one study of men aged 55 to 59.

Coronary Heart Disease continued

The good news is that it appears as a person's diet is changed to reduce the amount of animal fat consumed, so the survival rates significantly increase. See the graph below:

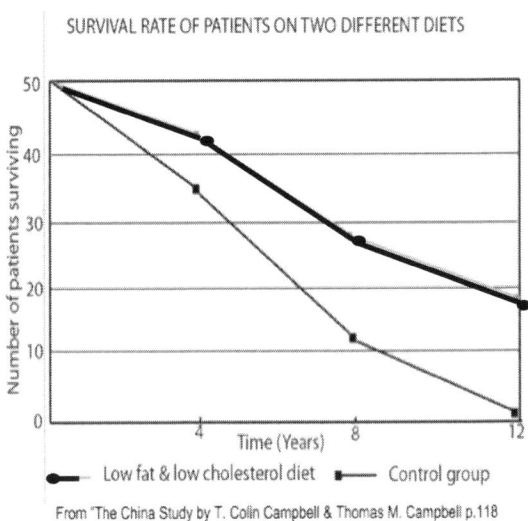

From "The China Study by T. Colin Campbell & Thomas M. Campbell p.118

Of fifty patients with a history of serious heart problems, 20 survived over 10 yrs who maintained a low fat, low cholesterol diet, *compared with only 5 in the control group eating their usual diet.* However it has now been discovered that it is not just animal fat consumption but also the animal protein that is involved in the increased risk. See graph below:

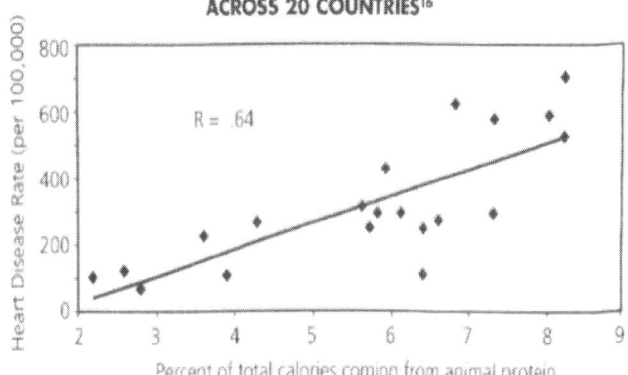

From "The China Study by T. Colin Campbell & Thomas M. Campbell p.120

Coronary Heart Disease continued

An eminent American surgeon, Dr. Esselstyn, was concerned about the poor treatment of cancer and heart disease as there was little effort at prevention as most research work focused on treatment. He began a major study looking at the effect of reducing fat and cholesterol intake of his patients. This meant almost eliminating all animal products, refined oils, dairy produce, fish and fowl. Of the group of patients that adhered to this dietary change, the average cholesterol levels fell from 246 mg/dL at the start to below 132 mg/dL. Over the 11 years of the study only one participant had a coronary event and this was a patient who had strayed from the diet for two years; after this incident he returned to the plant-based diet and ceased to have any symptoms or further events. Since Dr. Esselstyn's study similar results have been reproduced by others and all show the same dramatic improvement to the patient's condition and reversal of heart pathology in most cases. All patients who had agreed to angiograms showed reduced narrowing of the arteries supplying the heart.

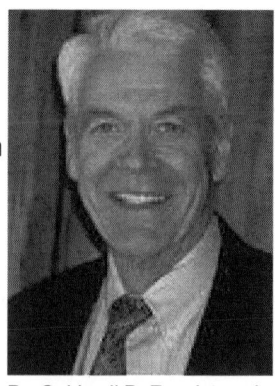

Dr. Caldwell B. Esselstyn, Jr.

Ref C1

Cateracts & Macular Degeneration

Of all our sensory systems, our eyes are perhaps the most affected by our general health and in particular by our dietary habits. Inadequate nutrition of specific essential nutrients has been shown to have a damaging effect on our eyesight, whether causing the accelerated development of cataracts or macular degeneration. The most important nutrients seem to be carotenoids that are readily available in a whole plant diet but are almost non existent in an animal based diet. Other antioxidents have a beneficial effect on our eyesight and what research has been done points to a very similar picture.

Overall it would seem that serious eyesight degeneration can be reduced by as much as 88% by simply eating a diet rich in anti-oxidents primarily found in a whole plant diet.

See the chart opposite, showing nutritional content of a whole plant based diet compared with an animal based diet.

Cateracts & Macular Degeneration continued

(PER 500 CALORIES OF ENERGY)

NUTRIENT	PLANT-BASED FOODS *	ANIMAL-BASED FOODS **	RDA
Cholesterol (mg)	-	137	0-?
Fat (g)	4	36	20-?
Protein (g)	33	34	50
Beta-carotene (mcg)	29,919	17	900
Dietary Fiber (g)	31	-	25
Vitamin C (mg)	293	4	90
Folate (mcg)	1168	19	400
Vitamin E (mg)	11	0.5	15
Iron (mg)	20	2	18
Magnesium (mg)	548	51	420
Calcium (mg)	545	252	1300

* Equal parts of tomatoes, spinach, lima beans, peas & potatoes. ** Equal parts of beef, pork, chicken & whole milk
Anti-oxidants

Ref C2

Diabetes

There are two types of diabetes; Type I, sometimes called juvenile onset diabetes, as this affects young children and Type II used to be termed adult onset diabetes. In the past decade the age classification has been dropped as children represent almost half of Type II diabetics now.
Type I diabetes is an autoimmune disease that usually incurs massive damage to the pancreas with an inability to produce adequate insulin.
Type II diabetes rarely shows such severe pancreatic damage and is responsive to dietary changes.
Repeated trials of low fat, high unrefined carbohydrate diet has shown marked improvements in both Type I and Type II diabetic patients.
The insulin dosage reduced by 40% to nil in some cases and the cholesterol levels showed a dramatic fall.
A second major "side-effect" recorded of those following a high carbohydrate, high fibre diet was a substantial fall in their cholesterol levels. See the charts on the next page:

Ref D1

Diabetes continued

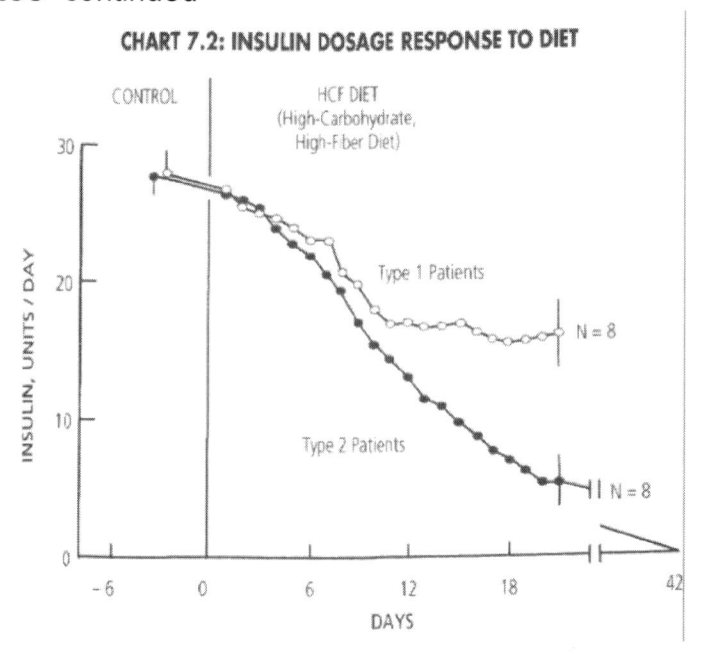

CHART 7.2: INSULIN DOSAGE RESPONSE TO DIET

From "The China Study" by T. Colin Campbell & Thomas M. Campbell p153

CHART 7.3: BLOOD CHOLESTEROL ON HIGH-CARBOHYDRATE, HIGH-FIBER DIET

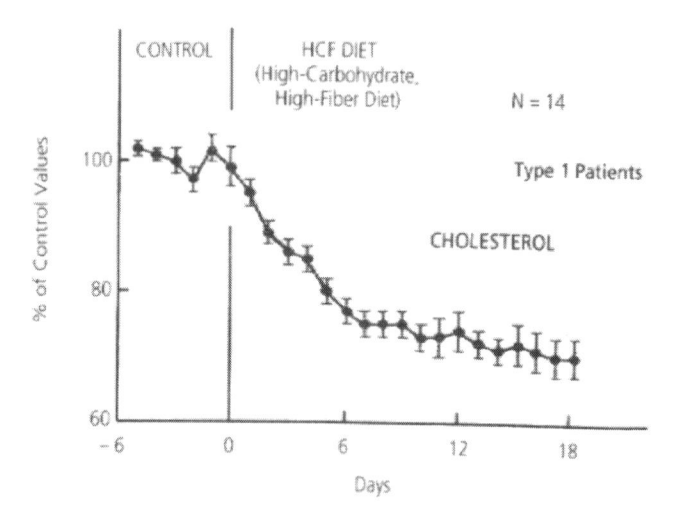

From "The China Study" by T. Colin Campbell & Thomas M. Campbell p154.

Diverticulosis

A condition rarely seen a generation ago but easily treated with dietary changes. *Inadequate fibre in our diets is the main cause of this modern disease.* Dietary fibre is found primarily in whole plant foods and not in animal based foods.

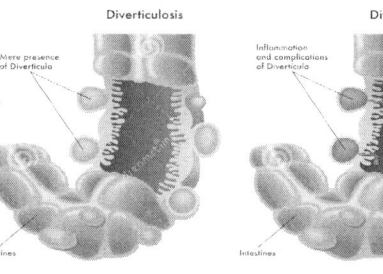

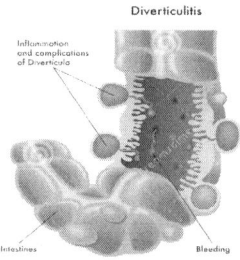

Without adequate fibre gut movement of content becomes very difficult requiring bowel straining and increased internal pressures that lead to the pockets of gut that may also become infected and inflamed creating a more serious condition, diverticulitis.

Ref. D2

Environment Destruction & Our Diet

Most animal based foods require many more times the water and energy input than the whole plant based foods. This puts a strain on the planet's ability to sustain such a diet; water resources are depleted, greenhouse gases are increased, tropical forests are destroyed, fossil fuels are depleted, further damaging the atmosphere, land erosion gets worse, waterways are polluted with run-off from artificial fertilisers. Heavier uses of herbicides and pesticides, essential to mechanised farming of these foods, increases the toxic load on us all and on the rivers and seas. Quite simply this process is not sustainable, and we must start to consider the future of our grandchildren in a world so damaged and depleted. See Environment Connection.

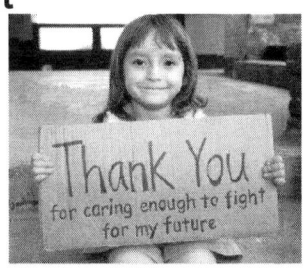

Ref. E1

Famine & Malnutrition

More than 870 million people in the world suffer daily from hunger. Every year, six million children will die from starvation. One third of all hunger victims can be found in developed countries, primarily a factor of poverty, as is the case with fifty million Americans. But the destructive forces of hunger often can be most complicated in developing countries where the other two thirds affected by hunger struggle to live, systemically impairing these nations health and progress in many ways. A shift towards a lower animal food diet globally could solve this problem with enough food for all.

Ref. F1

Gall Bladder Problems

There is a dietary connection between the development of gall bladder problems and consumption of animal based protein. You would never know you had a gallbladder unless it became filled with stones and angry, then you might find yourself rolling on the floor in agony – wishing you knew more about this little pear shaped sack attached to your liver's under surface and how to keep it healthy and happy. If your gallbladder acts up you are not alone. An estimated 20 million people have gallstones or have a history of surgery for gallstones in the United States. While most cases cause no symptoms, there are a half million gallbladder removals (cholecystectomies) and 800,000 people are hospitalized for gallbladder disease annually. Approximately 30% of Americans over the age of 60 years have gallbladder disease. Fortunately, serious symptoms and complications, such as inflammation, infection, pancreatitis, and bile duct obstruction, develop annually in only about 1% to 2% of patients. Gallstones are solid, rock-hard formations in the gallbladder made from crystals of cholesterol. The medical term for these is cholelithiasis. There is a saying for likely gallstone candidates, "female, fat, and forty." Gallstones are more common in women & in people who are over-weight. Over 90% of the gallstones found in Americans are considered cholesterol gallstones. For gallstones to be considered cholesterol stones, 70% to 90% of their material by weight must be cholesterol. Dr. John McDougall explains the connection between our diet and the development of gall bladder problems as primarily due to over-saturation of the bile with cholesterol. Cholesterol is only found in an animal based diet, so to avoid this problem, just cut back on the fatty oils and animal foods.   Ref.G1

Global Warming & Our Diet

Most of us are aware that our cars, our coal-generated electric power and even our cement factories adversely affect the environment. Until recently, however, the foods we eat had not been in the discussion. Yet according to a 2006 report by the United Nations Food and Agriculture Organization (FAO), our diets, and specifically the meat in them, cause more greenhouse gases; carbon dioxide (CO_2), methane, nitrous oxide, and the like to enter the atmosphere than either transportation or industry. Greenhouse gases trap solar energy, thereby warming the earth's surface.

Global Warming & Diet continued

Because gases vary in greenhouse potency, every greenhouse gas is usually expressed as an amount of CO2 with the same global-warming potential. The FAO report found that current production levels of meat contribute between 14 and 22 percent of the 36 billion tons of "CO2-equivalent" greenhouse gases the world produces every year.

Ref G2

Hypertension

Hypertension is often seen as a predictor of more serious health problems such as Coronary Heart Disease, a stroke or heart attacks. All the factors leading to heart disease affect blood pressure as well as chronic hidden hyperventilation usually arising from chronic stress. The evidence points to our diet being the key to this health problem & all that follows. Stress is perhaps the second most important factor behind hypertension & should always be addressed with some form of relaxation or stress management. Breath training has been shown to be an effective way of reducing the adverse effects of stress. For more information on the effect of stress & chronic hidden hyperventilation see "The Breath Connection".

Ref.H1

Kidney Stones

There is a dietary connection between the development of kidney stones and consumption of animal based protein that was researched over 50 years ago by Dr. W G Robertson. The chart below shows one part of his findings, that a small increase of animal protein from around 21 grams per day to 25 grams per day increased urinary calculi by 50%. He found by simply getting patients to shift from animal protein to all plant protein their kidney stone problems resolved.

CHART 10.4: ASSOCIATION BETWEEN ANIMAL PROTEIN INTAKE AND FORMATION OF URINARY CALCULI

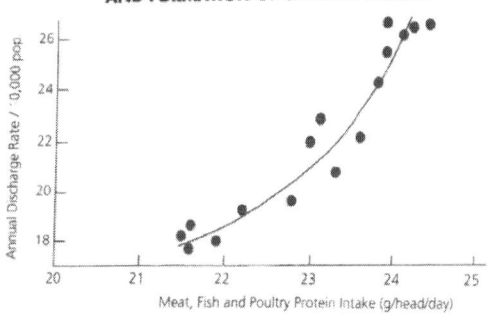

From "The China Study" by T. Colin Campbell & Thomas M. Campbell p213

Kidney Stones continued

The charts below show how the excretion of calcium and oxalates in the urine dramatically increase when any excess of animal protein is consumed. A further factor has also been shown to be involved, free radicals can trigger stone formation in the kidneys, as has been pointed out before free radicals are mopped up by anti-oxidants found only in a plant diet.

CHART 10.5: EFFECT OF ANIMAL PROTEIN INTAKE ON CALCIUM AND OXALATE IN THE URINE

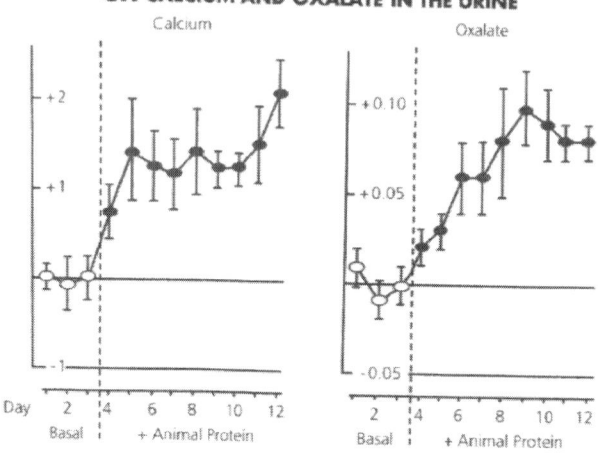

From "The China Study" by T. Colin Campbell & Thomas M. Campbell p214

Ref. K1

Liver Cancer

Major research with animal subjects has shown animal protein will increase liver cancer development once triggered by any carcinogen and that plant-based protein does not. Rats were given a known liver carcinogen, half of them were fed a diet of plant based protein, the other half were fed on an animal based protein. Every rat developed the expected liver cancer that had been given animal protein but none of the rats fed on plant protein developed cancer. The increased liver cancer development is related to the quantity of animal protein consumed. Reduction in animal protein consumed has the effect of slowing or stopping the cancer development. The cancer could be switched off and on by changing the level of animal protein consumed. The impact of animal protein on potential cancer development maybe implicated in humans as well. (See Breast Cancer & Animal Food Diet)

Ref.L1

Lupus

Lupus is just one of many autoimmune diseases that all have common features that include: A dysfunctional body immune system that attacks itself, they are more common in higher latitudes where there is less sunshine and consequently lower levels of Vitamin D, they tend to associated with other autoimmune conditions in the same people, all those diseases that have been studied for a nutritional connection show an association with consumption of animal protein, especially cow's milk, & there is evidence that a virus may trigger the disease. At this time there is no clear evidence from research that the above factors raise the risk of autoimmune diseases but there is a simple idea that some might agree with; if by changing our dietary habits and by carefully increasing our time in the sun there may be a beneficial effect of protecting us from these diseases, why not try this, if there are no risks from doing so? For those already afflicted with an autoimmune disease, a change of diet could be tried for a month or so and they could then ascertain for themselves whether or not they experienced any health improvement or reduction in symptoms. Nothing would be lost. There maybe another factor involved, your breathing or in particular your dysfunctional breathing arising from stress. To learn more about this see "The Breath Connection" section.   Ref. L2

Multiple Sclerosis

Multiple sclerosis MS has been an enigmatic disease. There has been no consensus of its cause or origins besides factors such as genetics, viruses and environmental factors but little attention has been paid to the role diet. Some of the earliest research on this concept was done by Dr. Swank in the USA. Remarkable long-term study of 144 MS patients involved the patient consuming a diet low in saturated fats. He classified patients as good dieters who maintained this restricted regime & those who strayed from the diet poor dieters. See the results in the graph above.

MS Death rate after 144 patients dieted for 34 years

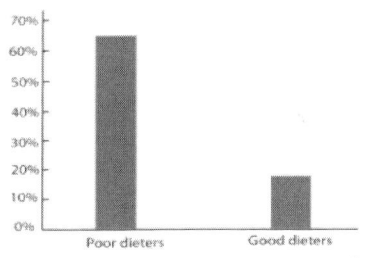

Chart 9.4 From "The China Study" by Colin T Campbell p196

Other studies have confirmed this association between cow's milk consumption and MS development. The graph on p.43 shows this by country.

Multiple Sclerosis continued

CHART 9.5: ASSOCIATION OF COW'S MILK CONSUMPTION AND MULTIPLE SCLEROSIS

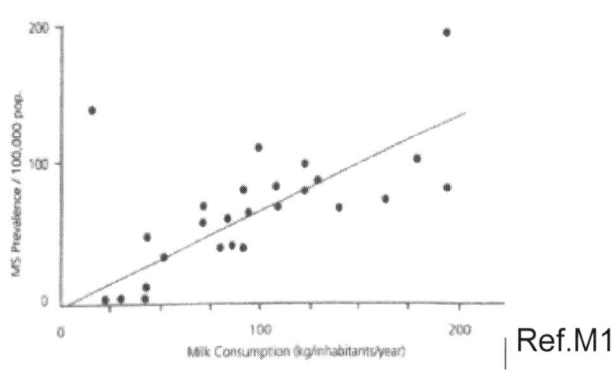

Ref.M1

Osteoporosis

CHART 10.1: ASSOCIATION OF URINARY CALCIUM EXCRETION WITH DIETARY PROTEIN INTAKE

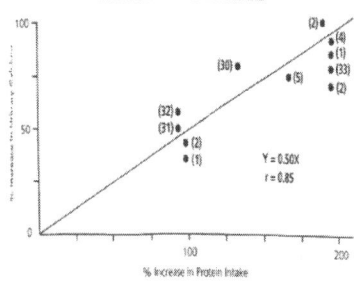

There is a well established belief that we should all consume a substantial quantity of dairy produce to ensure we get an adequate supply of calcium to protect ourselves from osteoporosis and the risk of hip fractures. This has been the official advice for over 50 years. The unfortunate truth is that all research suggests otherwise, in fact it appears the incidence of hip fractures, a good indicator of osteoporosis, increases with increased dairy produce consumption. This may be due in part to the fact that increased dietary protein (usually animal based) causes increased urinary secretion of calcium. See chart above.

The left axis shows %age Incresed Urinary Calcium excretion.
From "The China Study" by T Colin Campbell & Thomas M. Campbell p206.

CHART 10.2: ASSOCIATION OF ANIMAL VERSUS PLANT PROTEIN INTAKE AND BONE FRACTURE RATES FOR DIFFERENT COUNTRIES

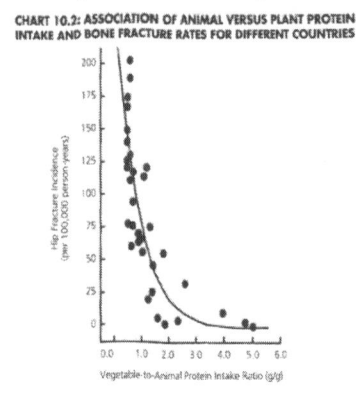

The second factor may be the impact of diet on hip fractures related to the proportion of animal protein to plant protein consumed, the lowest rates of hip fractures are found in countries with the highest proportion of plant based protein. See chart opposite.

From "The China Study" by T Colin Campbell & Thomas M. Campbell p207.

Osteoporosis continued

Finally, the belief that the higher our calcium intake, the lower our hip fractures does not prove to be true. See chart opposite. All these contradictions to established thinking are in part due to the complexity of calcium metabolism & lack of good quality research. This research has not been well received by the dairy industry who's repeated advertising promotes increased dairy product consumption, to produce strong bones. When we look at the comparative calcium content of animal based foods versus plant based foods, the reality is that *plant based foods contain twice the calcium as animal based foods.* Ref.O1

Chart 10.3: Association of Rates of Hip Fractures with Calcium Intake for Different Countries

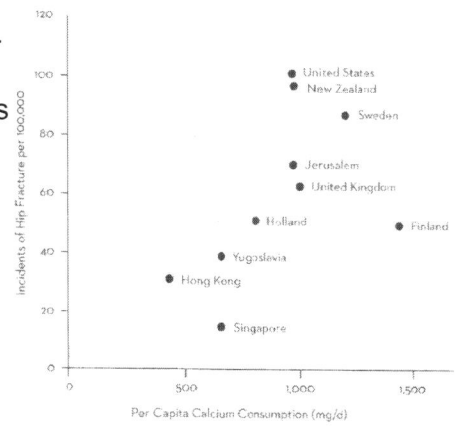

Prostate Cancer

The key factors associated with the development of prostate cancer are:
1. Prostate cancer rates vary widely between different countries.
2. High prostate cancer rates primarily exist in societies with Western diets and lifestyles.
3. Those men from developing countries who adopt Western eating habits or move to Western countries suffer more prostate cancer.

The relationship is: *a plant-based diet is associated with lower rates and an animal-based diet with higher rates of prostate cancer.*

The most specific link between diet and prostate cancer is dairy food consumption. This association may be related to higher intake of calcium & phosphorus. There is a hormonal link; a hormone our bodies produce as needed, namely Insulin-like Growth Factor1 or IGF-1, appears to be as good a predictor of prostate cancer as cholesterol is for heart disease. Studies show men with higher than normal levels of IGF-1 have a fivefold risk of advanced stage prostate cancer. An added risk factor is due to low levels of vitamin D. Vitamin D is produced by the body when we are in the sun and the production of the highly activated vitamin D is controlled by our body. This process is conditional on what we eat & animal protein tends to block the production of supercharged vitamin D and persistently high levels of calcium reduce vitamin D production.

Prostate Cancer continued

Lower levels of this supercharged vitamin D can lead to prostate cancer. The commonest animal-based protein that contains substantial calcium is dairy produce.

Rheumatoid Arthritis

Rheumatoid arthritis is just one of many autoimmune diseases that all have common features that include:
1. An Immune system that attacks "self" proteins as if they were foreign.
2. They are generally in higher latitudes where there is less sunshine.
3. Found together with other autoimmune diseases in the same individual.
4. All diseases studied in relation to nutrition, the consumption of animal-based foods, especially cows milk, is associated with greater risk.
5. There is evidence that a virus may trigger the onset of many of these diseases.
6. The mechanisms of action of these diseases have much in common. Inadequate sunlight exposure, consumption of animal-based foods, especially cow's milk, and low levels of vitamins D all seem to be factors. At this time there is no clear evidence from research that the above factors raise the risk of autoimmune diseases but there is a simple idea that some might agree with; it by changing our dietary habits and by carefully increasing our time in the sun, there may be beneficial effects protecting us from these diseases and if there are no risks why not try? For those individuals already afflicted with rheumatoid arthitis a change of diet could be tried for a month or so and they could then ascertain for themselves whether or not they experienced any health improvement or reduction in symptoms. Nothing would be lost. Ref.R1

Stroke

In a famous study, The Framingham Study, researchers found that for every three additional servings of fruit and vegetables per day the risk of a stroke was reduced by 22%. Increasing the proportion of vegetables and fruit in our diets not only offers increasing protection against strokes but protection is given against vascular dementia or Alzheimer's disease because of healthier arteries. Surely here are two good reasons to start altering our diets? Stress can also play a part in the development of this disease, read "The Breath Connection" section on this subject. Ref. S1

Weight Problems
Creeping weight gain has been a problem as affluence develops. The chart below shows the vast changes since 1978 in various countries.

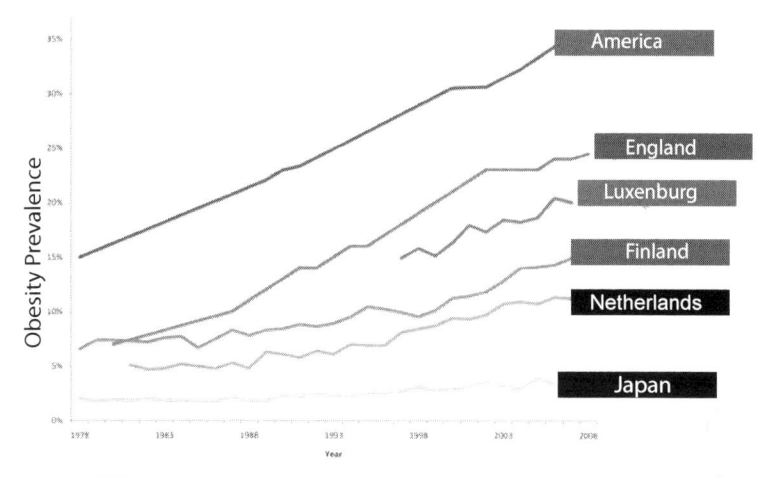

Source: OECD http://www.ecosante.org/index2.php?base=OCDE&langs=ENG&langh=ENG
*Self reported data (prevalence rates for the other countries are based on measured data)

The solution is relatively easy and it doesn't mean starving yourself! Eat a low fat, whole plant based diet & enjoy a moderate amount of exercise. A number of studies have shown significant weight loss from following such a diet varying from 2 to 5 pounds over 12 days to 24 pounds over a year. However other factors are involved such as how overweight the person who starts the diet, not eating refined carbohydrates, doing adequate physical exercise & the particular metabolism or body type of the person. This relationship could be seen in the China Study where rural Chinese ate far more calories per pound of body weight but were slimmer than their American opposites.

Dietary Q & A's (Destroying the old myths on diet)
Q1. How does our diet affect our cholesterol levels?
A1. An Animal Based Diet (ABD) will give a higher intake of cholesterol versus a Plant-Based Diet (PBD) *since practically no cholesterol in plants*.

Q2. Do we need meat to ensure we get adequate protein?
A2. Protein *content is the same for both* ABD & PBD

Q3. Can we get enough iron from a plant based diet?
A3. A PBD *gives ten times more iron* than an ABD   continued.......

Dietary Q & A's continued

Q4. Should children be fed dairy produce to ensure they get sufficient calcium for growing bones?
A4. *Calcium content is doubled with a PBD and essential magnesium is ten times higher with PBD*
Q5. What level of antioxidants can be found in a animal based diet?
A5. Anti-oxidants (vitamins) negligble quantity in ABD *our principal source of anti-oxidants is from PBD*
Q6. Will we get adequate fibre in an animal based diet?
A6. *No fibre in an ABD* more than RDA in PBD. Fibre is essential for healthy digestive functioning & healthy gut flora.
Q7. Is it possible to live a healthy life just on plants?
A7. The only potential deficiency is B12 and possibly Vitamin D if living in northern climates or severely protected from the sun.
Here supplements may be advisable but not always necessary. If in doubt have your doctor arrange a blood test to establish your situation.
Q8. Is it easy to change ones diet so radically?
A8. No! But don't try to change overnight, take it in small stages and don't stress about it. If you believe it is worth the effort from all the evidence, then start to make your food your the most delicious and health promoting medicine ever prescribed! "Let food be your medicine & source of joy!"

The nutritional content of 500 calories of both a plant based diet & an animal based diet are given in the table below. It is given here again as it is a great reference base to answer many of the questions you may have yourself or be asked by friends and family. RDA is the official recommended daily allowance for a healthy diet.
Most of those questions are answered by reference to this data.

NUTRIENT	PLANT- BASED FOODS *	ANIMAL-BASED FOODS **	RDA
Cholesterol (mg)	-	137	0-?
Fat (g)	4	36	20-?
Protein (g)	33	34	50
Beta-carotene (mcg)	29,919	17	900
Dietary Fiber (g)	31	-	25
Vitamin C (mg)	293	4	90
Folate (mcg)	1168	19	400
Vitamin E (mg)	11	0.5	15
Iron (mg)	20	2	18
Magnesium (mg)	548	51	420
Calcium (mg)	545	252	1300

* Equal parts of tomatoes, spinach, lima beans, peas & potatoes. ** Equal parts of beef, pork, chicken & whole milk

More Information on Whole Plant Diet

Forks over Knives Cooking <http://www.forksoverknives.com>

McDougall's Health & Medical Centre <https://www.drmcdougall.com>

T. Colin Campbell Center for Nutrition Studies <http://nutritionstudies.org>

Prevent & Reverse Heart Disease <http://www.dresselstyn.com/site/>

Nutrition Facts <www.NutritionFacts.org>

The Physicians Committee for Responsible Medicine <http://www.pcrm.org>

Engine 2 Diet <http://engine2diet.com>

Preventive Medicine Research Institute <http://www.pmri.org/index.html>

The Plant-Based Dietitian <http://plantbaseddietitian.com>

Plant-Based Docs (The Plantrician Project) International Directory <http://plantbaseddocs.com/>

Forks Over Knives – Over 230 plant-based recipes! <http://plantpoweredkitchen.com>

The Wellness Forum - <http://www.wellnessforum.com>

TrueNorth Health Centre <http://www.healthpromoting.com>

Books

The Starch Solution – Dr. John McDougall   ISBN 978 -1-62336-027-6
Prevent and Reverse Heart Disease Cookbook by Anne Esselstyn ISBN 978-1-58333-558-1
The China Study by Drs. T. Colin Campbell and Thomas Campbell. ISBN 978-1-932-10066-2
The Forks Over Knives Plan Drs. Alona Pulde & M Lederman. ISBN-13: 978 1 47675330 0
Let Them Eat Vegan by Dreena Burton. ISBN: 978- 0-738-215617
The Happy Herbivore Cookbooks by Lindsay Nixon ISBN 1 0 19356 1 8121
The Breath Connection by Michael Lingard <www.lulu.com/spotlight/lingard>
How Not To Die by Dr. Michael Greger ISBN 978-1-4472-8244-0
Whole - Rethinking the Science of Nutrition Dr. T Colin Campbell ISBN 978-1-937-85624-3
The Campbell Plan - Whole Plant Based Diet Dr. Thomas Campbell ISBN 978-1-62336-410-6
Dr. Neal Barnard's Program Reversing Diabetes - Dr. Neal D Barnard ISBN 978-1-59486-810-8
The New McDougall Cookbook - Dr. John McDougal & Mary McDougal   ISBN 0-525-93610-6
Full Planet, Empty Plates - Lester R Brown   ISBN 978-0-393-34415-8
Forks over Knives The Cookbook - Del Sroufe   ISBN 978-1-61519-061-4
Dr. Dean Ornish's Program for Reversing Heart Disease - Dean Cornish ISBN 0-394-57565-2
The Pleasure Trap - Douglas J Lisle   ISBN 978-1-57067-197-5
The Complete Idiot's Guide to Plant-Based Nutrition by J Hever ISBN978-1-61564-101-7

See <http://www.thefoodconnection.org.uk/betterhealth.html> for more practical recipe advice.

The Breath Connection

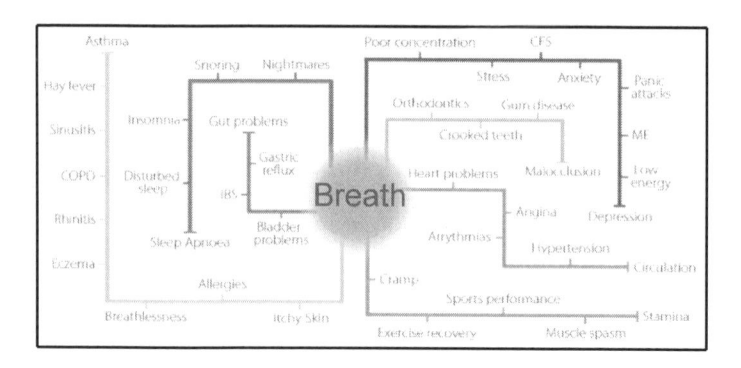

1. Breathing is vital for life
We can go for weeks without food, days without water but only minutes without air. Perhaps then we should pay more attention to our breathing?

2. Stress makes us breathe more because of the fight/flight reaction, any stress increases our breathing. Repeated stresses can lead to chronic hidden hyperventilation.

3. You can have too much of a good thing. Over-eating leads to obesity & serious health problems, we can effectively drown if we drink too much water, and too much breathing also has serious damaging effects on our health.

4. Over breathing makes you ill. Professor Buteyko claimed that over one hundred and fifty modern diseases are associated with over-breathing, the most common being asthma, sleep apnoea, hypertension and panic attacks.

5. Most of us habitually over-breathe. The majority of us in the West suffer some degree of chronic over-breathing. Either it is the chronic effect of our stressful lifestyles or perhaps in part due to a culture that promotes deep breathing in exercise classes, in gyms and whenever we are stressed we are told to "breathe deeply"

Summary of the facts: We, like all mammals, are given about 500,000,000 breaths in a lifetime: learn to use them well. It is without doubt the most important activity in our lives & yet it is almost totally ignored in medicine unless there is some respiratory pathology. Stress triggers increased breathing and chronic stress creates chronic hidden hyperventilation that leads to poor health or serious illness.
The good news is, we can all correct this bad habit with just a little effort.

Normal Breathing

Your doctor checked your blood pressure, your weight, your reflexes, your blood chemistry, your heart & lung sounds, you may have had Peak Flow tests, even given you X-rays or MRI scans but why didn't he check your breathing rate?
That seems strange, doesn't it?

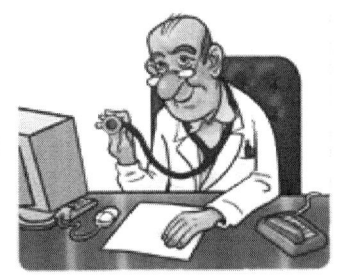

That life's most fundamental activity, BREATHING, is not routinely checked by Western doctors (unless you are complaining of breathing difficulties like asthma, COPD or bronchitis) is a serious omission. If there were just one measure allowed when checking the health of a person I would suggest THEIR BREATHING would be the best choice. Why?
Firstly it's a quick, easy and cheap test. It takes less than a minute, is none invasive and does not require special expensive equipment.
Secondly, many medical researchers have claimed dysfunctional breathing may be the cause of over a hundred modern diseases, so wouldn't it make sense to at least diagnose it and then perhaps address this problem first?
Thirdly, although our breathing is normally automatic and unconscious - like our heart, liver, & kidney activity - we *can* take conscious control of it and change our bad breathing habits for good normal ones, with just a little training.
Fourthly, this route to better health and wellbeing empowers the patient and reduces their reliance on medical care and drugs. Surely a very desirable aim?

Normal breathing is defined as a gentle respiratory action of 8-10 breaths per minute, through the nose, using the diaphragm not the upper chest. This action moves 4-5 litres of air per minute through the nose, in and out the lungs.
This maintains the optimal chemistry of the body, with a normal range of pH & with 40mm partial pressure of CO_2. If our breathing increases CO_2 levels are reduced and all body chemistry is adversely affected & as the nose cannot easily cope with this volume of air we begin to mouth breathe.

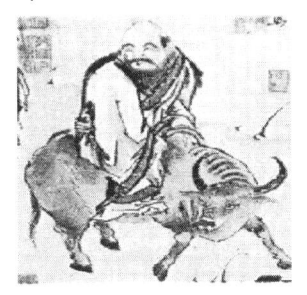

Two thousand years ago a wise man said:
"The perfect man breathes
as if he is not breathing."
- Lao-Tzu (circa 4th century BC).

What Controls our Breathing?

There is a sensor in the medulla of the brain that monitors the level of CO2 in the blood. As soon as the CO2 reaches the point where the brain detects an abnormal level of the pH, the brain activates the diaphragm and breathing is increased or reduced to correct this.
We don't need to concern ourselves with our breathing, it's automatic, but it can go wrong!

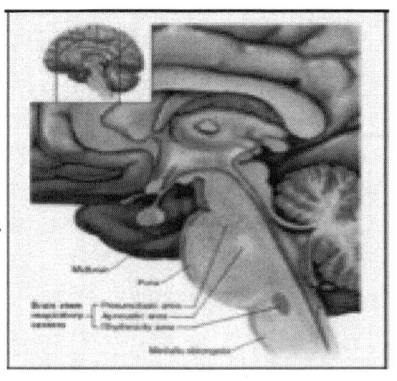

Why is CO2 so important?

Carbon dioxide is not only vital for all life on this planet but is the prime controller of many vital functions in our bodies. If the CO2 level falls too low & remains so, many chronic illnesses may develop. CO2 is involved in the following processes:

1. It controls our breathing.
2. It prevents spasm of smooth muscle wrapped around blood vessels, airways, gut, bladder etc. throughout the body.
3. It activates the release of oxygen from the blood into our cells for normal functioning. (The Bohr Effect)
4. It maintains normal range of pH (acidity/alkalinity) of the blood to optimize all body chemistry.

If the CO2 levels fall too low any of the following problems can occur:
Breathing becomes disordered, the person may be locked into hyperventilation as the receptors in the brain accept a lower CO2 level.
Smooth muscle throughout the body starts to spasm.
Asthma attacks may occur in those genetically predisposed.
Sinusitis & other upper respiratory tract problems may be triggered.
Digestive disorders such as gastric reflux & IBS may develop.
Circulatory problems, typically hypertension (high blood pressure) may occur.
Spasm of bladder can cause disturbed sleep & urinary frequency.
Impaired oxygen release from the blood (The Bohr Effect) impairs all cell functioning, regeneration or energy conversion.
Poor sleep and excessive tiredness may be experienced during the day.
Skin disorders such as eczema can develop.
When CO2 loss is severe at night, the body shuts down breathing to conserve CO2, this is one of the major causes of sleep apnoea, (the cessation of breathing while asleep for long periods).

Do you have any of these symptoms?

If you tick more than three or four of the following symptoms you could be a dysfunctional breather and would benefit from a breathing retraining course or at least it would be sensible to have a breathing assessment.

Allergies
Angina
Anxiety
Apathy
Asthma
Bad breath
Bed wetting
Belching or Flatulence
Bloating
Breathing without pause
Chest pains (not heart)
Cholesterol elevated
Constipation
Coughing
Cramps (muscle or gut)
Dental problems/deformities
Depression
Deterioration of vision
Diarrhoea
Difficulty in swallowing
Digestive problems
Disturbed sleep patterns
Dizziness
Dry mouth
Eczema/other skin problems
Excessive mucus production
Excessive yawning or sighing
Flashes before the eyes
Fluid retention
Frequent deep breaths
Gastric reflux
Haemorrhoids
Hay fever or rhinitis
Headaches

High blood pressure
Insomnia
Irregular heart beat
Irregular or painful periods
Irritability
Irritable bowel syndrome
Kidney problems
Loss of concentration
Loss of libido
Loss of memory
Loss of smell
Mental fatigue
Mouth breathing
Muscle pains
Night-time toilet trips
Nose bleeds
Numbness around lips
Orthodontic problems
Pains in the bones
Palpitations
Panic attacks
Ringing or buzzing in ears
Shortness of breath
Shuddering in sleep
Sinusitis
Sleep apnoea
Snoring
Sweating
Thyroid problems
Tightness of chest
Trembling or tics
Varicose veins
Weight gain or loss

Why is Hyperventilation not Easily Noticed ?

Most people cannot believe they hyperventilate because they do not show any dramatic outward signs. Just think, if you breathed 7-8 litres per minute instead of the normal 5-6 litres/min, no one would notice. If you breathed slightly faster than normal you could add another 2 litres/min. unnoticed and if you were to sigh or yawn every few minutes this could add another 2 litres/ min. The overall effect of these minor changes in your breathing habits could lead to you breathing 10-15 litres of air per minute instead of the normal 5-6 litres per minute in other words *two or three times normal.*

History of Professor Konstantin Pavlovich Buteyko

Konstantin Pavlovich Buteyko was born near Kiev in Russia on January 27th 1923. This simple yet extraordinary man devoted his life to studying the human organism and made one of the most profound discoveries in the history of medicine. Prof.Buteyko commenced his medical training in Russia in 1946 at the First Medical Institute of Moscow. Part of one of his practical assignments involved monitoring the breathing of terminally ill patients prior to death. After hundreds of hours spent observing & recording breathing patterns, he was able to predict with accuracy the time of death of each patient. Each patient's breathing increased as their condition deteriorated and as they approached death.

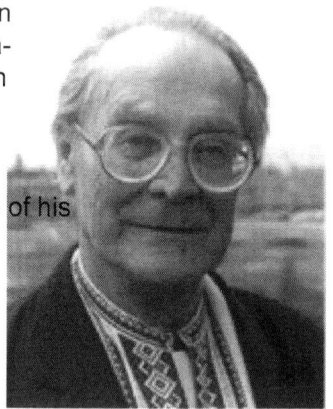

While at University, Buteyko was diagnosed as suffering from malignant hypertension. This is a fatal form of blood pressure which gave him life expectancy of just twelve months. By using his new-found observations, he was able to bring his breathing back to normal levels and enjoy a further 50 years of life with a normal blood pressure. He did not appreciate it at the time, but this was one of the greatest, although as yet largely unacknowledged, medical discoveries of the twentieth century. Buteyko established that breathing, so vital in sustaining life, can be not only the cure but also amazingly the cause of so many of diseases of modern civilisation. It took until the early 1980's for his discovery to be recognised in Russia where it is now in common use in many Russian hospitals. It was brought to Australia in1990 by Buteyko & Sasha Stalmatsky, one of his teaching assistants in Moscow.With hundreds of Buteyko Educators thoughout the world the Buteyko Method is beginning to be internationally acclaimed.

Stress & The Breath Connection

Emotional, financial, housing, relationships, work, school, illness, family, environment, food, injuries, accidents, job loss, loneliness, travel, infections, pain, fear, anger, toxins, drugs, etc.

Stress

Health Problems

Allergies / Angina
Anxiety / Asthma
Breathlessness
Cardiac problems
COPD / Depression
Eczema / Epilepsy/tics
Chronic fatigue syndrome
Gastric ulcer / Headaches
Gut problems / Hay fever
Heart problems / Hypertension
Hyperthyroidism /IBS
ME / Migraines
Orthodontic problems
Rhinitis / Sinusitis
Sleep apnoea / Snoring

Fight/Flight Response

Increased Muscle Tension
Increased Mental Tension
Increased Breathing

Up to 1,400 physiological changes including: Impaired immune response / Increased blood volume from spleen / Release of steroid hormones / Release of stress hormone cortisol / Release of catacholamines / Increased secretion of adrenalin / Release of neuropeptides / Increased heart rate / Decreased fertility or adverse effects on pregnancy / Increased fat deposition & cholesterol levels / Increased blood pressure / Increased histamine production / Spasm of smooth muscle around vessels / Increased sleep disturbances / Increased inflammation of digestive tract / Reduced blood flow to skin / Impaired immune response / Increased / blood clotting reaction / Increased blood sugars etc./ etc.

It is well recognised that stress is a major factor in most modern diseases. With relaxation & breathing exercises we can reduce stress and its many adverse physiological effects.

The Breath Connection Training Courses

The correction of bad breathing habits that may have been present for many years cannot usually be achieved by reading a book or from a video but requires the individual supervision and skill of an experienced practitioner to recognize the breathing patterns and give the necessary support and advice to effect permanent changes.

Every person's breathing problem is unique and the training is tailored to meet these individual needs.

The Breath Connection training is usually tailored to the individual's lifestyle & time availability, it can be based on a series of Skype lessons at any distance, a one to one training course to fit in with the individual's work/time constraints or as part of a small group over two three hour sessions. All training involves monitoring and follow-up support for as long as needed to establish the changed breathing habits. It is also possible to give basic training of children in large groups within the school.

The Buteyko Method & Clinical Trials

The most extensive research into the effects on health of breathing was the life's work of Prof. Buteyko & much of this early work is being published on the internet. There have been a number of clinical trials that have substantiated the relationship between chronic hidden hyperventilation & asthma. More research is needed for other hyperventilation related conditions.

The Mater Hospital Trial Brisbane 1998

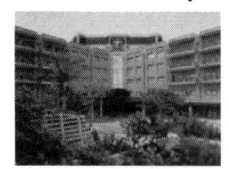

"Those practising the Buteyko Breathing Technique reduced hyperventilation and their use of beta2-agonists. (Reliever medication) A trend toward reduced inhaled steroid use and better quality of life......" For full details of this trial visit any of the Buteyko websites.

The Gisborne Trial New Zealand 2003

"The magnitude of effect in both studies was remarkably similar to the Mater trial, 85% reduction in reliever medication & 37% reduction in steroids." For full details of this trial visit any of the Buteyko websites.

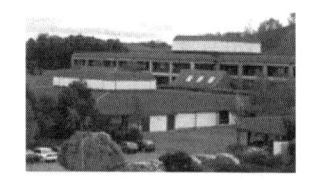

The Calgary Trial Canada 2007

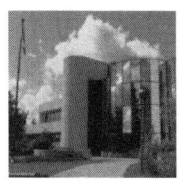

"I've been astonished and also very pleased with the excellent result. There is no disruption of their life at all by their disease: normal activities; not waking at night; not needing to use any reliever medications. It's just great...75% control is about as good as anyone has got in any study of asthma. The neat thing about it is that it has no side effects. It's very safe. The Buteyko technique certainly has been shown to be an important adjunct to treatment."....Dr. Robert Cowie Respirologist. For full details of this trial visit any of the Buteyko websites.

Asthma

Asthma is probably one of the most over diagnosed and over-medicated illnesses in the Western world. It is referred to as a "disease" which means that it is quite acceptable to keep on prescribing medications to control it. It is in fact NOT a disease, rather a condition that can be managed. The most popular treatment for this debilitating condition is inhaled reliever medication to relieve breathlessness, and steroid preventer medication to reduce inflammation and symptoms and reduce reliever usage. Little attempt is made to look at the root cause of the problem and to take steps to eliminate or manage the cause. Several research programs have been undertaken recently by non-aligned medical scientists whose research grants come from academic funding. However the vast majority of research is funded by the pharmaceutical industry who have no interest in any alternative approach to asthma management that requires fewer drugs as this would have a serious effect on their profits. Asthma drugs account for approximately 20% of their income.

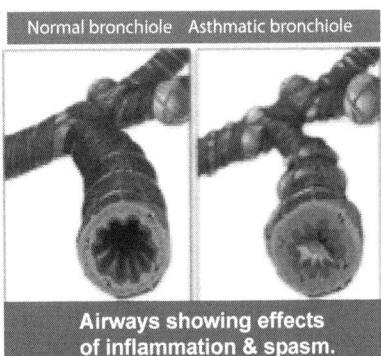

What the independent researchers have found is of great concern, and in a report released on the 17th June 2004, by the Cornell Institute, together with researchers from Stamford University stated clearly that the on-going use of beta-agonist relievers (such as Ventolin) can actually make asthma worse and can also be a causative factor in heart disease, heart attacks and even death. It is well known that people with asthma breathe far more than usual, are mostly mouth-breathers and gasp and pant when they have an attack. Most asthma reliever medications increase the breathing rate and make the problem worse, as CO_2 levels drop and airways go into spasm. Steroid preventer medications have a many side-effects which very often cause people to stop using them, thus putting themselves at severe risk from using reliever medication alone. Asthma medication has NEVER cured asthma, and those suffering from it usually use more and more medication as each year goes by. There are now new combination medications being widely prescribed. They are increasingly potent, and longer lasting. People are confused into believing that they no longer require their Reliever medication, unaware that Reliever medication is actually built into the new combination puffer.

Visit **<www.TheBreathConnection.com>** to download a leaflet on asthma and the way breath training reduces symptoms and need for medication.

Emphysema and COPD

Once lung tissue has been damaged it is not possible to regenerate it. The major problem faced by people with emphysema COPD is a is chronic shortness of breath as well as side-effects from the large amount of drugs they usually take. They also often suffer from a build up of mucus, usually aggravated by hyperventilation and excess histamine release. By learning how to breathe correctly, it is possible to reduce the amount of medication used thereby reducing the side-effects. It is also possible to increase the efficiency of the remaining lung tissue by providing it with the correct levels of CO2 and preventing spasm from occurring.

Most people with emphysema are often on several puffers, as well as a nebuliser, long-acting reliever & sometimes supplemental oxygen. Many of the long-acting puffers that are prescribed in high doses, for a long period of time, actually reduce the elasticity of the breathing tubes. (If you blow up a balloon, then let it down, blow it up again, let it down again, the walls of the balloon will become floppy and weak.) Those with emphysema who have done the Buteyko Breathing Programme have found that they are able to reduce their intake of medications, walk further, have far less breathing problems, and are sometimes able to do away with their nebuliser and enjoy a far better quality of life.

Eczema

Eczema is commonly found associated with asthma & other breathing problems. It is also very often found in people who are stressed. The skin is the largest organ of the body and is the furthest away from the heart. It therefore stands to reason that it will be the last to receive its supply of oxygen - which is required to build new cells to replace those that die.

If the cells are already dead, then it makes no sense to rub steroid and other creams into them. This will not bring them back to life. On Page xx we explained the Bohr Effect and the importance of CO2 in releasing oxygen from the blood. It therefore makes sense that if someone has perpetually low CO2 levels then they will have less oxygen available to build new skin cells. Hyperventilation is usually associated with increased secretion of histamines that further aggravate the skin problem.

Allergies, Sinusitis & Hayfever

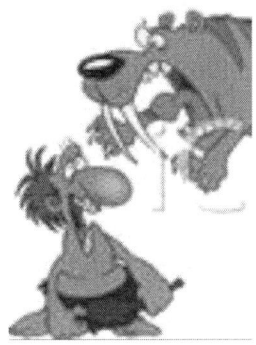

The human body is kept safe by a primal mechanism known as Fight or Flight. When the body perceives a danger, it makes a rapid decision whether to stay and fight, or to run away. In all cases of Fight or Flight, the first reaction is a shot of adrenalin to the bloodstream and this sets off a chain of other reactions which vary according to the degree of danger. Adrenalin, a stimulant that increases the breathing rate, so whenever we are stressed, we will breathe faster. This usually means breathing through the mouth, and this is when the carbon dioxide levels are lowered.

Whenever anything enters the human body, be it through the mouth, nose, eyes or skin, & the body is not comfortable with this substance, it will try to get rid of it. The reaction is usually to coat the offender with mucus or other secretions and then try to expel it. This explains why we sneeze, cough, vomit, develop a diarrhoea or break out in angry, itchy bumps or welts. Every one of these reactions is accompanied by the release of adrenalin and/or histamine and/or other chemicals which cause our breathing to rise. This rise in breathing rate lowers CO_2 levels and this causes more body stress.

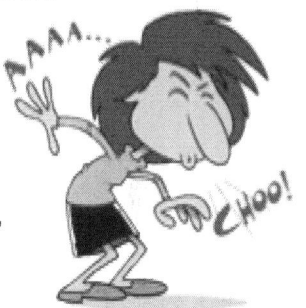

If this becomes chronic, such as with hay fever, rhinitis, sinusitis, coughing, sneezing and other allergic reactions, our breathing rate will be constantly increased, the CO_2 levels will drop and the brain will alter the trigger point, as previously explained.

When breathing is normal we can cope with higher levels of allergens. When our breathing becomes dysfunctional, we become overly sensitive to these triggers & they affect us at a far lower concentration than would normally cause a problem.

Constant coughing and sneezing lowers the CO_2 level even further and the condition becomes worse with more spasm in the smooth muscle in the nose, throat and lungs. Gasping and deep breathing actually make the problems worse, and should be avoided at all costs.

Snoring

Snoring is a major problem for millions of people. There are numerous "cures" on the market but very few of these address the cause. They prefer to try to manage the result, as this generates a great deal of money on an ongoing basis. Snoring can best be described as moving too much air over the loose tissues in the throat and nose, causing them to rattle. (The Venturi Effect)

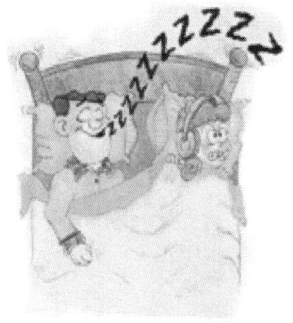

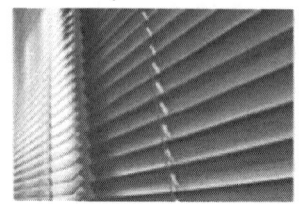

When a window is closed the blinds or curtains don"t move. When the mouth is closed during sleep, and when the volume of air moving in and out of the lungs is at the correct level of 4–5 litres per minute, the tissues of the throat & nose don't rattle and make noises.

So the most sensible way to address the issue of snoring is to try to re-establish breathing through the nose, rather than through the mouth and adjusting the amount of air breathed in and out, so that it falls within the normal limit.
There are other issues involved, such as being overweight and drinking too much. These are all stresses of one kind or another that contribute to the problem of over-breathing and are discussed on the Breath Training course.

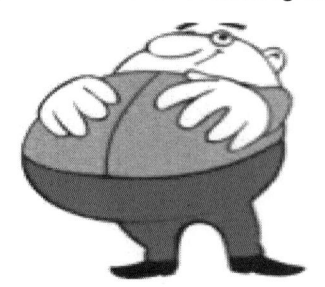

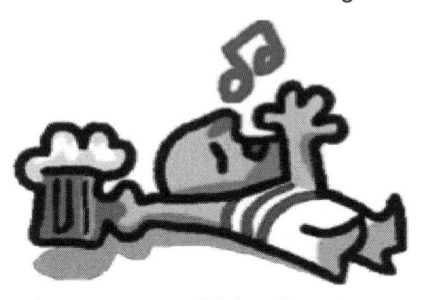

The answer is to learn a breathing exercise program which will restore your breathing through your nose and reduce the amount of air moving through the mouth and nose. As the airflow reduces, so does the noise, as the loose tissues in the mouth, nose and throat no longer "flap in the breeze" .
Recent research also suggests snoring may be a precursor of more serious health problems such as heart disease and sleeep apnoea. Download a pdf with more information on this subject from the Breath Connection website <www.thebreathconnection.com>.

Sleep Apnoea

Sleep Apnoea is one of the most frequently accessed topics on the Internet. Hundreds of thousands of people spend each night hooked up to machines to help them breathe. This has now reached epidemic proportions and sleep clinics are appearing everywhere as people desperately look for an answer to this debilitating problem.

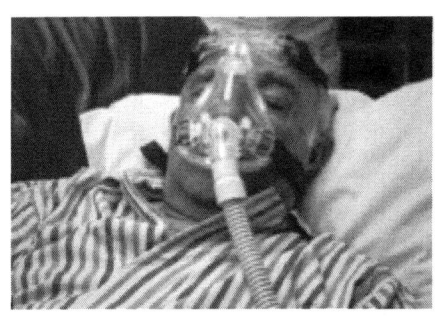

It is not only very large people with lots of loose tissue in the backs of their throats who have this problem. Many small and slim people suffer as well, and there are several reasons why this occurs. Some are physical and some chemical. Others are a combination of both and need a combination of approaches to achieve the result. On Page xx we discussed the importance of CO_2 in maintaining the correct pH of the blood. As soon as the brain detects that the CO_2 level is dropping to a dangerous level, usually as a result of heavy snoring or mouth breathing, it sends a message to the diaphragm instructing it to stop. Breathing then stops, the CO_2 level rises and the brain allows breathing to start again. The next breath is usually a gasp, which lowers the CO_2 level again and the process is repeated. There can be up to 40 – 60 such stop-start or "apnoea" events an hour and this is why people are constantly exhausted and unable to function throughout the day.

Accident risks to drivers from sleep apnoea are generally agreed to be as serious as alcohol consumption.

This reaction of the body to low CO_2 is a scientifically accepted principle known as The Bohr Effect, first described by Danish Physiologist Christian Bohr in 1904.

This problem can often be solved simply by keeping the mouth closed during sleep, and allowing the CO_2 to rise. Often, is all that the CPAP machine does. This can also be achieved, at a far lower cost, and with less trauma, by restoring breathing to normal. Certain cases may require a combination of both techniques.

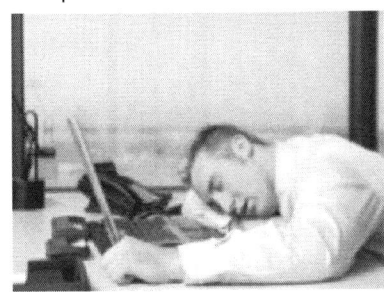

The Breath Connection can now offer continuous monitoring sleep studies to measure blood oxygenation levels, heart rate and frequency of apnoea episodes before and after breath training. For more detailed information download a free pdf from the Breath Connection website.

High Blood Pressure

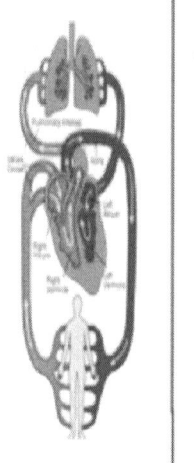

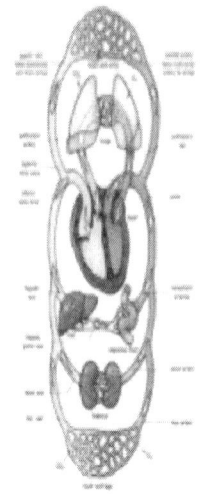

The body's circulatory system has around 100,000 km of various kinds of blood vessels. There are arteries, veins, capillaries, arterioles and other tiny vessels all of which are concerned with getting oxygen to body cells and bringing back excess CO2 and other by-products of metabolism. Look closely at the diagram below and you will see that each of the blood vessels has a layer of smooth muscle bands surrounding the tube. On Page xx we discussed the importance of CO2 in preventing smooth muscle tubes from going into spasm. If someone has low CO2 levels, their smooth muscle systems will be in a constant state of tension and constriction. In the circulatory system this leads to high blood pressure and it should be noted here that Professor Buteyko actually developed his breathing technique for himself in order to manage malignantly high blood pressure in his early 30's. By reducing the tension in his blood vessels by increasing his CO2 level, he bought himself an extra 50 years of life. Study stress & hyperventilation connection diagram on Page xx .

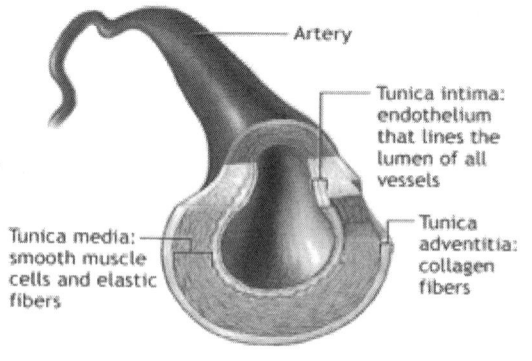

Learn how to control your breathing and lower your blood pressure the natural way. Clinical trials have proved that it is possible to lower blood pressure by a minimum of 14mm systolic and 9mm diastolic, by breathing at the body"s normal functional level. In the same way that spasm in the smooth muscle walls of the veins and arteries causes circulatory problems, so does spasm in the tubes in the digestive and breathing systems cause chronic health problems. All of the conditions on the symptoms list on Page xx have a direct link to dysfunctional breathing, low CO2 levels in the blood and the lungs, & the compromised release of oxygen from the blood.

Anxiety & Panic Attacks

It is thought that a high percentage of people suffer from some degree of anxiety and/or panic at some stage during their lives. This can be aggravated by some medications, pain, uncertainty regarding their health condition or life issues as well as past, present and/or future circumstances and situations. Some people live with this condition daily. Anxiety and Panic Attacks start the Fight or Flight response and the breathing rate automatically increases. As a result of this, the CO2 levels drop and the smooth muscle tubes throughout the body go into spasm. This is why people who suffer from these conditions often have difficulty in breathing, have stomach aches and pains, and generally feel less than well. Anti-depressants are sometimes required but in a large number of cases they are prescribed without addressing the cause of the problem & the side effects often make people feel even worse than they did before they started. The success rate for this problem has been very high as people learn to manage their anxiety with breath control. Mindfulness has become the current popular training which makes sense as much of mindfulness training is directed at normalising breathing.

General Health, Fitness Sport & Wellbeing

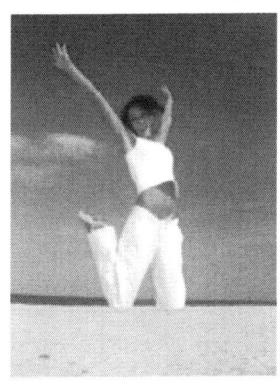

Many people are now choosing to do the Buteyko Breathing Course to improve their overall health and fitness. Because oxygen is so vital for good health, energy and stamina & because the release of oxygen from the blood is so dependent on the correct level of CO2 in the blood and lungs, you will be fitter, faster & more competitive if you learn to exercise with your mouth closed. You will also require less recovery time. You will have more energy and vitality, your memory will improve, you will sleep more restfully and generally enjoy a better quality of life. Many professional sports people have used the Buteyko Method for improved performance. **Why not give yourself the competetive edge over your rivals, whether in sport or in the cut & thrust of commerce, by better breathing! It stands to reason that if you ate or drank for two or three people, you would become chronically sick. The same applies to breathing for two or three people. At 30,000 breaths a day, it makes sense that even a small error in each breath, will add up to a major issue over a period of time. Oxygen delivery to the brain can be reduced by 50%.**

Dental & Orthodontic Problems
What has breathing to do with orthodontics? A reasonable question to ask! *So here's how you can prove the connection yourself.* First, breathe with your mouth open. Where is your tongue? Now breathe with your mouth closed. Where is your tongue now? Any dentist will tell you it only takes a pressure of a few grams to move a tooth, as this is how braces work. You will note that when you nose breathe your tongue pushes up on

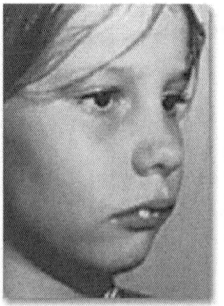

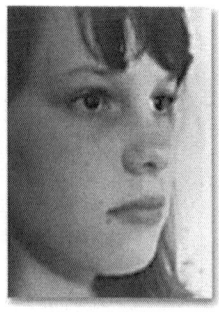

BEFORE (8½ years)   AFTER (12 years)

your palate. It is applying over 30 grams & this keeps the upper jaw wide and allows teeth to develop normally. If you breathe through your mouth all the time the palate can close up and cause the teeth to be crowded and irregular, a similar effect is occuring on the lower jaw but here another effect may be a receding jaw as well as crowded teeth. These orthodontic effects impact on the whole child's structural development & posture, not just the teeth!
Children and adults who mouth breathe *will* require orthodontic work. When your mouth is open, the tongue drops to the bottom, the cheek muscles continue to pull inwards but there is no opposing force from the tongue. The upper jaw then becomes narrow, the front teeth protrude and the rest of the teeth crowd. The palate becomes narrow and the vault rises and this often causes inflammation of the adenoids – resulting in infection of the upper respiratory tract. Unless the tongue is returned the correct position, against the roof of the mouth, there will never be long-term stability. In fact, it is generally accepted that about 90% of orthodontic work done will revert unless a retainer plate is worn permanently. Compliance with wearing retainers is very low, and this often causes friction between parents and their children. Many orthodontists recommend that no work be done until after puberty, but it makes far more sense to start early especially correcting breathing and prevent the problem from starting. *Mouth breathing can also cause: In addition to the structural effects described above, the onset of an asthma attack in those genetically predisposed, changes to the pH of saliva reducing its bactericidal value, inflammation of the adenoids, ear infections, often resulting in the insertion of grommets, coughs, colds and other respiratory infections and dry mouth and bad breath especially on waking.*

Visit the Breath Connection website for more comprehensive information & view the video By Dr. John Flutter on this subject. Tell your child "*They should breathe through their mouth as often as they eat through their nose!*" That will help!

The Breath Connection Training Course

What is Taught
Adults and children over five years of age are taught how to take better control of their condition naturally, training consists of the Buteyko Method & other lifestyle guidelines that have been proven to considerably reduce symptoms and reduce dependency on medication. All medication is continued alongside our programme but after a number of weeks practice of exercises & upon improvement of symptoms, medication may be reduced only after consultation with a medical doctor.

The Course includes:
Initial Consultation: To assess your condition. Registration & Introduction The History of the Buteyko Method the Science & Research.
Practical work: Nose clearing exercises, the Control Pause and Pulse measurement, Reduced breathing exercises, Sleep and breathing, Posture and breathing, Cough relief, Capnography to establish the severity of the problem, workbook for recording exercises, Refining the Control Pause, The Extended Pause, The Mini Pause, More Reduced Breathing Techniques, Talking & Nose Breathing Exercises, Food & Breathing, Food Testing, Controlling an asthma or hyperventilation attack, Pacing yourself, Review of Exercises, Review of Medication, Hyperventilation & its Effects on Health, Anti-Hyperventilation Exercises 1, 2 & 3 More Buteyko Exercises, Practical advice on Buteyko application, Understanding the Control Pause & Pulse significance, How to achieve a Control Pause of 35-45 seconds & above, Physical Exercise & Breathing, Sealing the Leaks, Breathing Awareness & More Buteyko Exercises , Do I need to see a doctor? End of Course Questionnaire, Review of Exercises, Exercise Reduction, Taking Physical Exercise, Warning Signs, Safe Medication Reduction, Buteyko & your GP, Golden Rules for Good Health "The Doctor's Guide to the Buteyko Method" End of Course Important Points, Final Capnography when indicated to assess overall changes in breathing function.

Fees:
This is a "once in a lifetime" investment in your health. The Breath Connection Course teaches you to replace bad breathing habits with good ones for a healthier life. Once you have completed the course you will have the skills taught you for life. You will not need to spend more time or money on learning to breathe better in the future but simply put these skills into practice on a day to day basis.The cost for the full programme depends on whether you attend in person, do the course on Skype, have a 1-2-1 or group course. Discounts for certain groups are always available, please ask about this, as it is our aim that no one should be discouraged from taking this training because of financial difficulties.

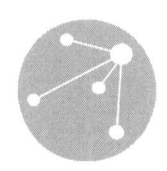

The Breath Connection
"Better Breathing Means Better Health"
Now Check Your Own Breathing

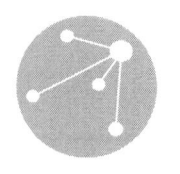

Did you know almost 90% of the general population in the West over-breathe, in other words suffer from some degree of chronic "hidden" hyperventilation. Hidden hyperventilation has been shown to be associated with over a hundred complaints from simple fatigue to hypertension and asthma.

Check your own breathing here. You will need a second hand or stopwatch for timing yourself.

Sitting comfortably, make sure you are breathing quietly and normally for a minute or two, through your nose. Keep the mouth closed, and on an out-breath, lightly nip your nose and hold your breath until you feel you want to breathe again, release the nose and ensure you return to normal depth and rhythm of breathing immediately afterwards. You shouldn't need to take a large in-breath or deeper breath, *if you do, you have held your breath too long*. Time the duration of this breath hold. **This is your Control Pause (CP)**, the number of seconds you can comfortably hold your breath after a normal out-breath.

Check below to see how good your breathing is:

Your CP	Breathing	L/Min	CO_2	Degree of hyperventiltion
45-60 sec.	Excellent	4-5	6.5%	Normal healthy breathing
35-45 sec.	Good	6-7	6.0%	Mild over-breathing
25-35 sec.	Fair	8-10	5.5%	Significant hyperventilation
15-25 sec.	Poor	10-12	5.0%	Serious hyperventilation
10-15 sec.	Very poor	12-15	4.5%	Very serious hyperventilation
5-10 sec.	Critical	15-20	4.0%	Hyperventilation at critical level

The above figures are approximate values but we can check your actual alveolar CO_2 level with our Capnograph and we usually have additional assessment measures including the Nijmegen Questionnaire, Haemaglobin oxygen saturation and where necessary sleep studies.

If your CP is under 20 seconds it is most likely your breathing is having an adverse effect on your general health and you should make an effort to improve it before you develop chronic health problems. Check out the Breath Connection Training Course options on our website.

Doctors Comments Worldwide

"The simple fact is that 34 patients, prior to Buteyko, were costing £15,000 for their asthma medication," he said. "After Buteyko, they were costing £5,000. That's a reduction of two-thirds in their drugs bill. If this was extended to the rest of the country, very significant savings could be made."
Doctor Gerald Spence Glasgow UK

"The ability to produce marked reductions in asthma drug utilisation suggests that the pharmaceutical economic implications of BBT (Buteyko Breathing Technique) merit further study. Clarification of the mechanism(s) underlying the effectiveness of BBT is a further goal, given that BBT appears to represent a safe, efficacious alternative for the management of asthma."
Dr Patrick McHugh, Emergency Department, Gisborne Hospital, New Zealand et alia

"The Buteyko Institute Method provides a comprehensive approach to achieving safe and effective asthma control. I find that the Buteyko Institute Method helps control asthma through simple breathing exercises and asthma education, rather than medication, the method respects the doctor-patient relationship, teaching patients to control their reliever medication, only stepping down steroids under medical supervision. This is in line with accepted 'best practice' asthma management worldwide." Dr Anand, MBBS MRCGP, Newcastle upon Tyne UK

" I've been astonished and also very pleased with the excellent result. There is no disruption of their life at all by their disease: normal activities; not waking at night; not needing to use any reliever medications. It's just great...*75% control is about as good as anyone has got in any study of asthma. The neat thing about it is that it has no side effects. It's very safe.*The Buteyko technique certainly has been shown to be an important adjunct to treatment."
Dr Bob Cowie MD, MB ChB, MSc, FCP(SA) MFOM - Clinical Trial of Buteyko Method, Calgary Canada

"Those practising Buteyko Breathing Technique reduced hyperventilation and their use of relievers. A trend toward reduced inhaled steroid use and better quality of life was observed in these patients without objective changes in measures of airway calibre."
Drs Simon D Bowler, FRACP, Thoracic Physician.,Charles A Mitchell, FRACP, Assoc. Prof.

"Professor Buteyko's principles are entirely consistent with the physiological facts established by medical research 120 years ago. The Buteyko system makes use of the person's own resources & trains them in taking responsibility for their own health. They become less dependant on outside agencies such as hospitals, doctors and physiotherapists, reducing the costs to the health service".
Doctor Godfrey Nelson M.B.B.A, F.R.A.C, G.P UK

"Over the last two years I have examined many patients before and after the [Buteyko] course and found the improvement to be repeatable to the degree that patients in over 90% of cases can stop medical treatment, or reduce it to less than half, of that, which was previously required. I attended the tutorials and found the approach, tuition and the method to be responsible and safe. As a doctor and Naturopath, I am impressed and surprised at the effectiveness and safety of this natural approach..."
Doctor Paul Ameison, MBBS, MD, DAC, ND, UK

With such testimonials from Doctors and Respiratory Specialists as above there can be no doubt about the safety and efficacy of the Buteyko Method.

Patient Testimonials

"Really helped to reduce my medication, feeling much better. Normally two to three attacks per week, since the course I have been able to overcome all attacks with Buteyko." William G. Iden Green, Kent

"My asthma was getting worse before the Buteyko course. I've been able to overcome most attacks, my energy has increased, my appetite lessened, I have less tension. My condition has greatly improved. I was slightly skeptical about the course but now I am a firm believer, it works!" Lisa B. Sandhurst, Kent

"Much calmer, less likely to panic, have stopped getting sleep apnea. No reliever for three months now, down to one puff preventer per day (down from two to four), sleeping better, over-coming most asthma attacks, energy levels up." Vivien B. Wadhurst, Kent

"Wished I'd come across the technique forty years ago." Minimal reaction now to dogs that would previously trigger chest tightness immediately. Unaffected now any change in air temperature, this used to be a trigger. Great result!" David R. Dover, Kent

"My energy has increased and my health has greatly improved. Everyone should have the opportunity to do this course to optimize their health & wellbeing" Pamela F. Chislehurst, Kent

"I began to notice the benefits within a matter of days. As an asthmatic, after seven days Buteyko has already changed my breathing, asthma, sleep and has reduced my appetite, it really does work!" Daniel R. Bodiam, Kent

"I would thoroughly recommend the Buteyko technique to anyone wishing to be in better control of their asthma. Reduced use of Ventolin, prior to the course my condition was getting worse, now overcoming attacks, sleeping better, energy increased, less tension, greatly improved."
Carol R. St Leonards, East Sussex

"Stopped all reliever medication, condition greatly improved, less mucus production, clearer nasal passages, little or no coughing., sleeping better, energy levels increased" Dudley C. Headcorn, Kent

"Very pleased with my progress, no reliever needed, no chest tightness, no rattles, no snoring & breathing better." Judy A. Ashford, Kent

The above are just a few of the hundreds of thousands of people across the world who have found remarkable relief from their suffering with the Buteyko Method training. The great news is that they achieved these results themselves once they had learned the science and physiology of breathing and had trained themselves to breathe better.
The list of doctors commenting in this booklet are just a few of the hundreds throughout the world who have recognised the potential value of the Buteyko Method. **Why not ask your own doctor if he/she has examined the Buteyko Method & given it a trial in his/her own practice, if not, why not start now? Suggest he/she checks some of the research information or contact us & we will send him or her a free copy of the "Doctor's Guide to Buteyko"**

The Breath Connection & Technology

Capnography & the CapnoTrainer

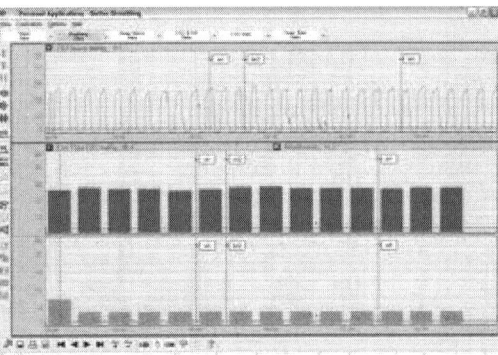

Capnography has been added to the Buteyko Method training programme with The Breath Connection to provide a more precise clinical record of changes in breathing chemistry before and after training. This will clearly demonstrate the changes in carbon dioxide levels due to improved breathing habits. In addition, data on heart rate, breathing rates and heart rate variability may be recorded. The second reason for the use of the Capnograph is the valuable aid to breath training offered by the CapnoTrainer. As can be seen on the screen shot here a live real time graph of a patient's CO2 can be observed & recorded whilst there is a moving image for the patient to track with their breathing. By adjusting the pre-set breathing rate and pause time between exhalation and inhalation patients can be challenged to modify their breathing pattern in order to return their breathing to normal. It is hoped that such additional clinical recordings will help substantiate the effectiveness of this training method & thereby encourage the use of such screening routinely for hyperventilation and the introduction of the Buteyko Method for its correction into NHS practices.

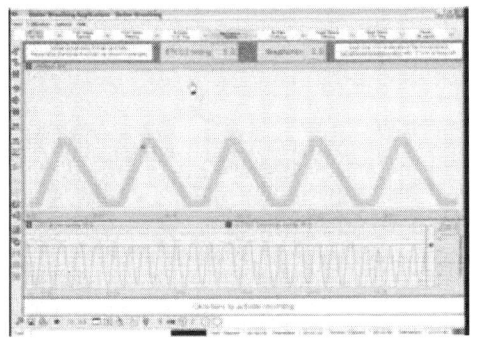

The Capnograph provides a totally non-invasive assessment of alveoli carbon dioxide concentrations and the heart rate data can give an insight into the working of the autonomic nervous system, the balance between sympathetic & parasympathtic activity.

Summary

1. Better breathing improves our general health, gives sound sleep, less tension and better digestion.
2. Better breathing boosts oxygenation of all the body's tissues; our muscles, our nervous system and the entire metabolism.
3. Better breathing safely reduces the need for medication, whether for asthma, hypertension, panic attacks, gut problems, hay fever or many other conditions.
4. Better breathing for children reduces the need for orthodontic work and the risk of poor structural development.
5. Everyone can learn to breathe better for life, with only a few days training and a Buteyko Educator in just a few weeks and change a lifetime's bad habit.

The Mind Connection

The Plastic Brain

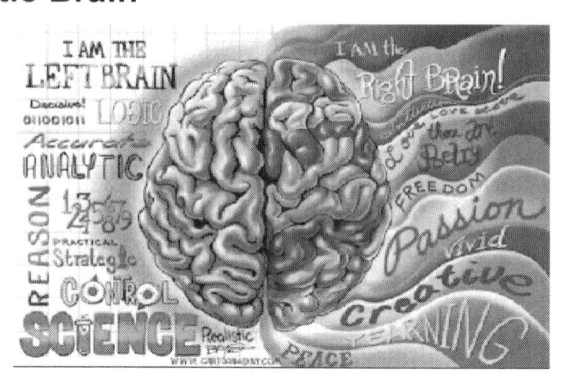

The most amazing thing about the human brain is that it has the ability to grow, change, rearrange all our thoughts and mental processing from birth to death. We have a plastic brain that can do remarkable things such as cope with a stroke and re-organised all the activities that were done in one area that is damaged and allow them to be done in another area. Areas of the brain that are normally associated with speech can be used for sight or hearing.
The old thinking was that we were born with a brain divided up into little boxes, each was allocated a specific job, this has all changed with the latest research. What does this mean to you and me? The first lesson we need to learn is never to say never! We cannot tell what is possible and what is not possible. The second lesson is that we can change the way we think, feel or behave in remarkable ways with a little help and effort. The third lesson is that despite the fact that we function much of our waking time with habits learned since childhood (it would be tough to have to learn how to talk, walk or clean our teeth the new every day!) all these habitually programmed activities can be reprogrammed. How we can do this is the subject of this section of the book. The phrase used today is "If it fires, it wires!" Repeated nerve signals create stronger pathways.

The Plastic Brain - How can we change it?

There are many aids that can be used to effect changes in the brain. All of us experience such changes throughout our lives without even being aware of it because at the basic level this happens automatically, as when we learn a new skill such as learning to play a musical instrument or a game of tennis. Areas of our brain that are needed to process this new information will expand and grow. Sometimes the reverse may be true, if we cease to do learned activities the corresponding areas of our brain will shrink.
Support and help to facilitate this process of change can be give with many therapeutic techniques such as Neuro Linguistic Programming or NLP, Hypnotherapy, Mindfulness, Emotional Freedom Technique or EFT, Counselling and many others. In addition such changes can be made by anyone themself,especially with determination and effort on their part.

Did you also know that every child at birth has a greater potential intelligence than Leonardo da Vinci ever used? That includes your own children and grandchildren. This is the subject developed later in this book that is based on many years of clinical research and practical application with tens of thousands of babies by Dr. Glen Domam and others. [36]

Finally, remember your mind is closely linked to all of the body activities and is perhaps the most significant connectiveness discussed in this book. We are emerging from a long period of study and thinking based on reductionism, or the analysis and study of increasingly smaller and smaller parts of our whole, but now there is a move towards the more difficult task of understanding how every part is connected to every other part and every system is affecting every other system, this is Holism or Wholism.

Neuro Linguistic Programming - NLP

NLP is an explicit powerful model of human experience and communication. Using the principles of NLP is possible to describe any human activity in a detailed way that allows you to make many deep and lasting changes quickly and easily. However it is only a tool and although it may be successful with one person in one situation, it may not be the appropriate tool for another person in a different situation. There are few tools that work for everyone in every situation.
Here are a few of the possible outcomes that NLP has made possible:

1. Cure phobias and other unpleasant feeling responses in less than an hour.
2. Help children and adults with "learning disabilities" (spelling and reading problems, etc.) (these limitations, often in less than an hour.
3. Eliminate most unwanted habits - smoking, drinking, overeating, insomnia, etc., in a few sessions.
4. Make changes in the interaction of couples, families and organisations so that they function in ways that are more satisfied & productive.
5. Cure many physical problems - not only most of those recognised as "psychosomatic" but also some that are not - in a few sessions.

Remember NLP may achieve many of the above things but it cannot do everything. If NLP fails to work it is the practitioner's responsibility to find another way.
Neurolinguistic programming is all about communication, how we communicate with ourselves and how we process communication (verbal and non-verbal) within the world with people around us.

NLP, along with other tools is used to help people find their goals and enable them to make decisions that will improve their lives and get the very best out of themselves by making better choices.

Hypnotherapy

Hypnotherapy is the use of hypnosis for therapeutic purposes.
The term hypnosis is used to describe a state of awareness dominated by the unconscious mind. Hypnotherapy can help with in many situations including :

Anxiety, stress and panic attacks.
Bereavement.
Confidence and low self-esteem.
Emotional issues.
Exam and test nerves.
Fears and phobias.
Habits (nail biting, skin picking, etc.).
Insomnia and sleep problems.
Migraines and pain relief.
Public speaking.
Relationship issues.
Smoking.
Stress management.
Weight control/ disordered eating.

Hypnotherapy is a natural, safe and effective way to make positive and beneficial life changes. With hypnotic techniques, old habits and patterns ofbehaviour can be changed, past hurts can be healed, negative beliefs can be discarded and much more can be changed to help you achieve what you want.

The word "trance" is just another term for hypnosis. When a person is in a trance or hypnosis they become more aware of their inner thoughts, feelings and sensations. This allows the conscious mind (critical, analytical mind) to be by-passed therefore allowing the creative mind (subconscious mind) to be more receptive to positive and beneficial suggestions.

Emotional Freedom Technique - EFT

EFT is a technique based on the meridian are system (similar to acupuncture but without the use of needles) and is capable of helping mental, physical and emotional issues. It was developed in the early 1990s by Gary Craig and works on the principle that " The cause of all negative emotions is a disruption in the body's energy system". By tapping on certain points on the face and upper body, blocks are released thereby allowing the "Chi" or energy in the body to flow freely again. Craig had studied Dr. Callaghan's Thought Field Therapy in the 1980s, an evolution of John Diamond's Kinesiology, both of which were rooted in ancient Eastern "meridian energy" theories of acupuncture and Shiatsu, codified since at least 1000BC.

EFT is especially effective in clearing traumatic memories: accidents, abuse, violence, childhood memories; or even clearing persistent negative messages from family or key people in our lives.

EFT has impressive results on a whole spectrum of emotional issues but is perhaps making its biggest impact on those suffering from post traumatic stress disorder.

Few therapies allow a patient to say aloud that they accept themselves despite their rape / abuse / addiction, while dealing with the emotions that arise simultaneously. With this approach people can change how they feel about something, but also accept that they can't change what happened –

that's the emotional freedom.

EMDR - Eye Movement Desensitisation

EMDR, (eye movement, desensitisation, reprogramming/reprocessing) is an innovative method of psychotherapy which has been used by trained mental health professionals to help an estimated half a million people of all ages from many different countries.
The focus of EMDR treatment is the resolution of emotional distress arising from difficult childhood experiences or to aid the recovery of critical incidents: car accidents, assault, natural disasters and combat trauma. Other issues treated with EMDR phobias, panic attacks and substance abuse, as well as performance enhancement - improving functioning of people at work, in sports and in the performing arts.
EMD and Reprocessing (EMDR) is a psychotherapy treatment that was originally designed to alleviate the distress associated with traumatic memories (Shapiro, 1989a, 1989b). Shapiro's (2001) Adaptive Information Processing model posits that EMDR therapy facilitates the accessing and processing of traumatic memories and other adverse life experience to bring these to an adaptive resolution. After successful treatment with EMDR therapy, affective distress is relieved, negative beliefs are reformulated, and physiological arousal is reduced. It enables people to heal from the symptoms and emotional distress that are the result of disturbing life experiences. Repeated studies show that by using EMDR therapy people can experience the benefits of psychotherapy that once took years to make a difference. It is widely assumed that severe emotional pain requires a long time to heal. EMDR therapy shows that the mind can in fact heal from psychological trauma much as the body recovers from physical trauma. More than 30 positive controlled outcome studies have been done on EMDR therapy.

Life Coaching

The average person has 60,000 thoughts every day and 95% of those thoughts are the same as we had the day before! This can subsequently create the same feelings we have about ourselves or the situation we are in. At times, life seems stuck and going nowhere, then all of a sudden, it's galloping out of control.

When we are stuck, we long for a change; when life is out of control, we want things to stay the same.

We experience change every day, as the world we live is constantly changing. We may change our hairstyles, the clothes we wear, the car we drive, our job.... But how often do we change the way we behave or react to events, or the way we feel or think?

Every interpretation, action & thought we make every minute has an effect on our mind and body. (***If neurones fire together they wire together***) **Here's the good news!** We can change those interpretations because we made them in the first place! We have the power to make choices. Just knowing this may be enough for you to make changes if you need to and want to.

Life coaching is a process that helps you identify and achieve goals by developing belief in your talents and skills to enable you to create the lifestyle you want.

Life coaching is not about looking into the past, but about where you are now - where you want to be and how you going to get there. Life coaching will give you the support and encouragement to get the results you want, whether it is in your personal or professional life.

Mind Myths & Facts

1. Hypnotherapy allows the therapist to take control of my mind.
Fact: Quite the reverse, hypnotherapy allows **you** to take control of your mind and the therapist helps you to have this for **yourself.**

2. Hypnosis is like having a general anasthetic, I'll be unconscious and not know what's going on.
Fact: When we are in a hypnotic state it is like the daydreaming state we experience many times everyday. We are often not consciously aware of everything we do all the time, otherwise we would be overwhelmed

3. Stress is something we just have to learn to live with, as we can't do much about it.
Fact: We can learn ways to reduce the impact of stress on our lives by learning effective coping strategies.

4. I have always had a fear of "Spiders..Heights..Dogs.....", I don't think that can change.
Fact: Most of our fears can be based on an association experienced a long time ago that is not relevant to the fear itself. NLP & hypnosis are extremely effective in dealing with fears and phobias.

5. I have always had an addiction to "whatever", I can't see how I can change that. Old habits & patterns of behaviour are well established.
Fact: Our addictions or cravings are, in part a mind problem, that can be retrained to minimise the effect.

6. Hypnotherapy won't work for me as I know I wouldn't be a good subject for it.
Fact: It is rare for clients not to benefit from hypnotherapy with the right approach.

The Living Connection

This story began for the author with an eminent pathologist by the name of Dr. G. Scott Williamson who after a lifetime of experience studying and discerning the nature and origins of disease one day asked himself a simple question that would dominate the rest of his life. It would ignite a flame of enghtenment that is still burning strongly today despite the passage of over eighty years of time and the domination of reductionism in almost all medical thinking and practice. As an experienced pathologist of his day Scott-Williamson was well able to give a sound explanation of the aetiology of most diseases; that was his work, but when he asked himself *what was the aetiology of health*, he had no answer.

Was health simply what was left after you removed all the diseases, or was it far more than that? In an effort to learn more with regard to this question he began to search the medical libraries in the UK and abroad but could find nothing on the subject. It would seem the medical profession had been so concerned and focused on pathology that the question of "health" had been almost ignored.

This moment was the birth of a large scientific experiment that was later to be known as The Peckham Experiment that involved over a thousand participants over a period of over twenty-five years.

In 1935, the Pioneer Health Centre opened its doors in Peckham for the first time. This community health centre, set up by Doctors George Scott Williamson and Innes Pearse, was a unique study into the health of individuals, families and their community. Its findings have had an impact around the world on those seeking to improve health and wellbeing.

The Pioneer Health Foundation now exists to promote the legacy of the Pioneer Health Centre and to highlight the relevance and importance of the Peckham Experiment today in the 21st century. A book published in 1980 brought together the findings of these two remarkable doctors, entitled "Science, Synthesis and Sanity" - An enquiry into the nature of Living by the founders of the Peckham Experiment. They chose the word "Sanity" rather than "Health" because even then "Health" carried the idea of dealing with disease and sickness, its diagnoisis, management and cure.

What is Health?

Health is everyone's birthright; the pity is that so many lose it, the difficulty is to see how it can grow and be developed. In spite of our vast sickness services, national health insurance, school medical inspections, ante-natal and post-natal clinics, welfare centres, tuberculosis and other clinics, the burden of ill-health in the community is heavy. Medical science advances rapidly with new treatments, drugs and instruments, but it does not seem to kill disease. So, quite logically, thought has turned to a more radical attack on disease: to protect people from disease and give them immunity. The preventative school is now at work on its plans. From the vanguard of this school another has emerged: those who believe that there is a negative ring in the words prevention, immunity and security; those who feel that it is a contradiction in terms to speak of protecting health, as though health were a weakling; those who believe that health is an active ' Positive ' thing, something as infectious as disease, which can also grow and spread. Such people speak of "positive health."

And there the track ends abruptly. For what is the nature of "positive health"? Out of what is it bred and how does it grow? Clearly bad economic conditions are enemies of this "positive health," but a study of those in the higher income groups suggests that they are not the whole story. We have had disease under the microscope. Our lenses grow more powerful. We see the cancer cell, the bacterium, and the body's scavengers. But the study of the nature of disease does not reveal to us the laws of health; it is health itself which we must study. We must devise a laboratory where we can study health, put it, too, under a lens, look at it, discover; how it behaves, and in what conditions it can grow and spread.

The above could have been written today but is an extract from a book, 'The Peckham Experiment' By Innes H. Pearse And Lucy M. Crocker. published soon after the second world war. Two potential ways forward were open to the healthcare in the UK at that stage, The Peckham Experiment based on Ethology or a Pathology based medicine. The latter was chosen and we now see the consequences.

The Experiment

The Peckham Experiment—the first laboratory in the world for the study of human health—began in the 1930's under the direction of two biologists, Doctor Scott Williamson and Doctor Innes Pearse. Research workers themselves, widely experienced in early diagnosis and in the investigation of disease, they had come to the conclusion that *no headway would be made in the cultivation of health by further research into the nature of sickness.* Intuitively aware that each person is born with an urge to health and a capacity for health that is seldom achieved, they sensed that health has its own pattern of behaviour, a pattern that is quite different from the pattern of disease. It was this pattern that they set out to study, and if you had asked them what they expected the Experiment to prove they would have told you " *that health is more powerful than disease.*"

The choice of Peckham as the site of the Experiment was the outcome of a careful search for a suitable area. Peckham had a mixed population. Pre-war wage levels rose from £20s.0d. a week (husband's income) to £1,500 or more a year. Small income people lived next door to the relatively rich, and a ten-roomed house might contain one family or be divided up to accommodate three. The bulk of Peckham people were sturdy families making their own way through life; they were free from gross poverty or continuous unemployment. Peckham was chosen as providing a cross section of low, middle, and upper middle income groups, and as likely to contain a maximum of people who might be presumed to be healthy.

These biologists started their work in a small house in Peckham, which they called the Pioneer Health Centre. Local families were invited to use it as a club. The member-families were offered through their club a periodic health overhaul. This gave the doctors their first opportunity to begin to study and assess health, while it gave member-families a chance of gaining for themselves modern knowledge to maintain such health as they had. The equipment of this small Centre was limited to a consulting room, an afternoon nursery for the children and a small club room. Here, mothers had a chance of meeting people over a cup of tea in the afternoons, and in the evenings both parents could enjoy a cup of coffee or a glass of beer, and now and then a whist drive or a concert.

Some First Conclusions

This was a small beginning, from which, at the end of three years' experimental work, the following facts were established: —

1. That there were families who welcomed and accepted the overhaul as a practical means of maintaining their health.
2. That the disorders which come before there is any definite disease can be thus detected long before the individual himself is aware that anything is wrong.
3. That disorders discovered in this early stage are much easier to deal with than in the later stage at which they are normally taken to the doctor.
4. Though the disorder, detected early, can usually be easily removed, with the cooperation of the patient, in a very large number of instances the disorder quickly recurs if the individual returns to the environmental conditions from which the disorder has sprung.

The general standard of vitality that they found, even in those who showed no early signs of disorder, was low. There was evidence of widespread inertia, of capacities unused, and with no outlet for expression, it was not poverty, nor any of the conditions that arise from poverty, for the families who joined the Centre were not in material want. Was there some inherent lack of vitality in the families themselves? They had money in their pockets, there was food for them to buy in the shops, yet they were not well nourished. There were swimming baths and tennis clubs in the borough, yet not even the young were well exercised. It was a crowded district and they had next door neighbours, yet they were isolated and friendless. They were, so to speak, hungry in the midst of plenty, and for no easily discoverable reason. Their vitality was low for want of things which were there for them to use & they did not use them.

Further Work Based on The Early Findings

The periodic overhaul had proved itself as a sieve for sifting out disease and disorder, but it was not, the doctors considered, by itself enough. Conditions seemed needed in which a family could find outlets for self-expression, in which it could recover vitality through a fuller use of its faculties. Doctor Scott Williamson and Doctor Innes Pearse decided to shut down the Centre and plan another. So the Peckham Experiment was now to be housed in the large, unusual & very beautiful concrete building, new both in structure and in concept, which was built to Doctor Scott Williamson's design—and to serve his special purpose—not by an Architect but by an Engineer, Sir E. Owen Williams. Money was raised for the purpose by a Committee, almost all of whom were young people. The money, lent and given came—in large and small amounts—from private persons. It should be made clear that those who subscribed did so in order to support a piece of research, and to make possible a social experiment of far reaching implications.

As well as the capital cost of the building, it was necessary to raise a development fund to pay for maintenance during the period in which membership was reaching the total of 2,000 families for which the experiment was planned. The family subscriptions and money spent in the club by adults (for all the children's activities were free) was estimated to cover running costs and ultimately to pay a small interest on capital. The War interrupted the experiment before membership reached the 2,000 mark, and so it was not then possible to demonstrate that such a service can be self-supporting, though there was evidence to indicate that this was a practical possibility.
The new building, was to provide a club for two thousand families, with a swimming bath, gymnasium, cafeteria (licensed to sell beer), a theatre, library, games rooms and nurseries. It was to supply them with a special kind of environment, an environment in which, moving freely, they could find wide and varied opportunities for action.
In the Centre they were neither directed nor organised, for health

must emerge spontaneously. The ' doctors ' were there to observe and to assess capacity not to mould people. They were there to study the ways in which health expresses itself. From this study they hoped to be able to formulate guiding principles for the cultivation of health.

It was a condition of membership that the member should be not an individual but a family unit, each family paying a subscription of one shilling a week, prewar. For this they had both periodic health overhaul and the use of the Centre's facilities. The Peckham families were independent, and "kept themselves to themselves " – " Oh, no, we don't know the people next door, we never speak to them." It was strange how rarely the young mother had any friends in the district, she had lost touch with her old school-friends or those she had made at work before she married. When she felt she needed company she went off to Fulham or Finchley to spend the day with her sister. The father was less cut off. He might drop in the local for a drink with a man met at work or on the train, or perhaps a game of billiards at the club, and on Saturday there might be a football match or an afternoon at the dogs. His wife, after the children came, could seldom go with him: there was no one she could ask to "mind the babies." When the children grew older, she did not even know the parents of the friends they made at school. There was no widening circle of friends coming into the home. In this isolation the family had lapsed into listless inactivity.

In the environment of the Centre they began to take hold of new opportunities. For instance, during the first three years after the second Centre opened, 157 married women, most of them middle-aged, had with no urging or persuasion—and very much to their own surprise— learned to swim. Out of 160 children between the ages of 5 and 16 who joined the Centre in 1937, only forty were swimmers. A year later, 128 of them could swim or were teaching themselves to do so. Opportunities which, though provided by the borough, had been ignored, were eagerly taken up in the Centre.

Now, and often led by the children, everyone was making friends. Out of swimming, dancing, the gymnasium, the theatre in which people acted, costumed and sometimes wrote their own plays, out of their own concert parties and orchestras, out of games, crafts and studies, making the teas for the babies in the nursery, and shared interests of many kinds, came new acquaintances and finally friends. Now , there were other families with whom the family was glad to go on holiday, with whom they could exchange impressions and ideas. The release from social loneliness & with it the increase in physical, mental and emotional energy was tremendous. This shift towards health and vitality was reflected in the findings at the yearly recurring overhaul of the family.

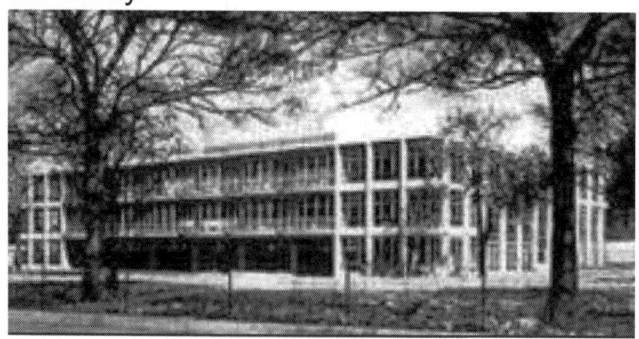

The Building Again

Since the Centre was built to the special design of the 'doctors' for the study of health, some description of its plan will help in understanding how the bringing together of these activities under one roof, and their careful adaptation to the leisure and needs of families came to make so distinct a change in the health of the family. The Pioneer Health Centre was built in concrete and glass. Its roof and its four walls, with wide bays on the side which caught the afternoon sun, were almost entirely of glass. In the centre of the building was the big swimming bath, the concrete tank of which occupied the depth between ground and first floor, its water level the level of the first floor, the sloping sides of its glass roof, through which swimmers could see the sky, rising above the flat roof of the rest of the building.

A glass band encircled the bath chamber and round this window was placed the cafeteria, where members could watch the swimmers. They could also look down on to the stage of the theatre, which was at one side of the swimming bath, and into the gymnasium which was on the other side. On the cafeteria floor there was also a large social hall. On the ground floor, as well as the gymnasium and the theatre, were the nurseries, changing rooms; and engine house. One side of the top floor was the only space shut off from general circulation. This was the consultation block with its laboratory, private consulting rooms, reception rooms and changing rooms. The rest of this floor was made up of large light open spaces for indoor games, for study, for a library, workrooms, wireless room, billiards, table-tennis, darts and whist, etc. Except where privacy was obviously essential, the partition walls were of glass. Visibility throughout the building of people and of their actions, was necessary for the scientists in this' the first "health laboratory." It gave them a special ' sight ' of their field of observation—the family. This transparency was their new ' lens.' Members were fully aware that whilst they were gaining from the opportunities which the Centre offered them, they were also contributing to the scientists' knowledge of health.

Sometimes one of the men would look at the doctors quizzically and say: " What are you getting out of this? " They got the true answer and were satisfied. But for the most part they were busied about in their own concerns and forgot about the 'doctors.' Natural, spontaneous and unselfconscious behaviour was a conspicuous quality of life in the Centre (visitors often commented on it) and indeed it was essential to the validity of the observations that this should be so.

The People Again
It will be clear that the design of the building itself invited social contact. It provided an environment for the chance meeting, for gala occasions as well as for acquaintanceship, companionship and for developing friendships, and also for the entertainment by families of visiting friends and relations. The activities which were taking place could be seen, and it was the sight of action which was the incentive to action.

Here it is necessary to stress two points. It is usually considered that it is the competent and skilled who are the incentive to action. That is true for those whose interest is already aroused, and who have some confidence and some pretention to skill. It is not true, however, of those who do not particularly want to do anything, who have no confidence and no skill. In the Centre it was found that the incentive to these—the great majority—was the sight of persons with less skill, who were even less well endowed with capacity than they. In the Centre there were people of all sorts doing all sorts of things, rather than small groups of experts doing things expertly to a large audience of spectators. In the Centre all eventually became 'doers.' The second point is that because the Centre was a family club, there were people of all ages mixing freely with one another as one does at home. That meant that there was always for the young a group just a little more mature than they—the people into whose company they naturally wanted to move. That in itself acted as a stimulus to them to grow. The adolescent wanted to be admitted to the group of young adults, so he strove to be, not only as skilled as they, but as socially competent as they. The young married couple without a baby, came to want a baby of their own like their slightly older friends, and so on. These natural stimuli to growth, and development can only emerge where all ages and types move freely in the general body of society. Any segregation into age and sex groups tends to confirm immaturity, and grading into select groups of experts tends to spectatorship of the mass rather than development.
The directors did not organise, suggest or promote any undertakings nor provide any 'leaders.' They discouraged members from forming themselves into permanent committees to organise their various enterprises. Thus there were no difficult thresholds for the new members to cross, no closed doors, no embarrassing applications, no cliques to intimidate the newcomer. There were, of course, difficulties, and there were a few people who behaved badly, but the community was finding its own way of dealing with any disturbing element. Members tended to live and to let live. They exercised their individuality in relation to each other, and it was found that individualism released from repression and operating in a mixed society cures itself of egotism. That is the basis of social health. The experiment was proving that in a suitable environment people will use the opportunities around them.

But what was perhaps more astonishing was the commonsense way in which they utilised new knowledge. Though communities may not respond to set teaching or to propaganda, and will resist persuasion, they will respond eagerly and purposefully to facts and information when they feel a use for them.

At Peckham

This spontaneous response of the ordinary man and woman to facts and information given objectively was a very early discovery. It had come out very clearly at the family overhauls in the first Centre, and it throws light on a very serious problem. Outside the Centre, people do not go to the doctor until very late, sometimes too late, but they went gladly to the Centre because they knew that they would be able to get full information in a form they could understand about "where they are and what they can stretch to"—as they put it. They knew that their overhauls were being made in order to find out what evidence there was of health and vitality, rather than as a search for what was wrong. So they never felt they were being made into 'patients.' Their overhaul was like a ship's survey at Lloyds — A1 at Peckham. "The 'doctors' tell you where you stand," they said.

There were two appointments for the overhaul: one for the laboratory and the other for the personal overhaul at which the father and boys were examined by a man, the mother and girls by a woman. When all the individuals had been examined the whole family met at a Family Consultation. The children were discussed one by one and then went out, leaving the parents with the two 'doctors.' Nothing was withheld in these talks. What was found in every member of the family was frankly reviewed; what it was, what it was not, and what it could be. No treatment was given and no advice, unless asked for. Every question—and there were many—was answered. Facts which doctors and specialists often consider too technical to discuss were as far as possible explained. The family was left in possession of the facts, free to use them as they thought fit.
The families went away and digested what they had heard; they thought it over and talked it over at home. They came to their own conclusions, and made their own decisions. If the decisions meant coming back and

asking for advice or help—if they wanted to get their teeth filled or had made up their minds to have a necessary operation, or to undertake some treatment—then the arrangements they asked for were made with their practitioner or with a suitable hospital or clinic. Every effort was made to make these arrangements to suit their own circumstances and their pockets, so that no one by looking after himself need expend unnecessary time or money, nor risk losing his job.

These consultations established a relationship between the Centre staff and the member-families from which both gained. Parents fell into the habit of discussing the way in which the family was growing up and the education of the children. The 'doctors' had seen the children in action in the Centre, as well as having examined them in the consulting room. From the correlation of these two sets of observations, as presented to the family by the doctors, the people often gained a fuller understanding of the way in which their children were developing. Husbands and wives discussed parenthood and whether or not to have more children. Most significant of all, young couples took advantage of the overhaul to achieve their fullest health before the conception of a child.

In the sample of society examined at their first overhaul in the Pioneer Health Centre, there were 10 per cent of individuals with nothing wrong, and roughly 20 per cent, who knew they had something wrong when they joined. The great middle group, which the biologists describe as being in 'well-being' because they would have spoken of themselves as being well, had some early disorder of which they were unaware or which they were ignoring. In the present state of society, this group inevitably drifts into disease, thus continuously swelling the number of the sick. In the environment of the Pioneer Health Centre, this large group, on the contrary, was tending to move towards health.

Finance.

The financial analysis of the Peckham Experiment suggested that such centres should be self-financing if members contributed (for all the family) approximately 2% of their income p.a. This today would be less than the membership of a modern gym or golf club for an individual.

Sanity.
Throughout the works of Drs. Scott Williamson and Innes Pearse the word "health" was purposefully avoided for good reasons.
The word "health" is derived from Anglo Saxon English "haelph" that in turn was derived from the root "hal" as in whole, hale & holy. The original word denoted a positive wholeness that has been lost with the passage of time & the rise in the science of pathology, so that today it has become synonymous with a lack of disease. This would infer that:
(a) That health is to be achieved by the fight against disease.
(b) That as diseases are cured and/or prevention has been achieved health will result.
We have been confused by the mis-use of the word consistently, calling "sickness services", "health services". That the real meaning of the word - wholeness - should be associated with the application of all the medical interventions of a multiplicity of drugs, surgery and monitoring devices, would seem not merely a semantic error but a serious and grave disaster for the real health and wellbeing of the nation. Today we have in the UK perhaps one of the best "sickness services" in the world but one of the poorest "health services".
It is interesting to note that many of us look at the world around us and feel we are living in an insane world in so many ways. Our observation is close to the truth when we replace "in-sane world" with an "un-healthy or a sick world".

Ethology & Pathology
What this work has demonstrated is that there are two distinct paths of study that are founded on quite different assumptions:
In the 1930's there was no scientific study of Health but a plethora of investigatrions of disease, little has changed over the past years to restore some balance in this area. Ethology is the study of health and all those factors that enhance or promote health whilst Pathology is the study of disease and all those factors that combat it. It is not possible to do justice to the work of these two doctors in this short article but interested readers should refer to the further reading references.

The Environment Connection

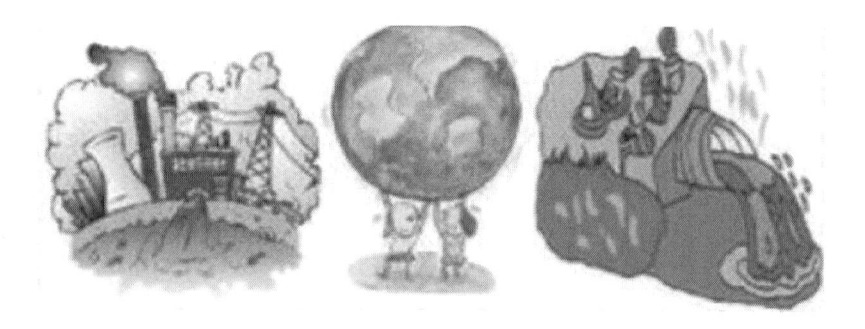

It would be impossible to discuss the health and wellbeing of an individual in any complete way without studying the impact of the whole environment upon them. This may, to many, seem a distant and almost irrelevant connection when viewed from their personal experience, but when we remember we all live on the same biophere we call earth. The places we live and work impact on our health through "the body connection", the earth's soil, oceans and water affect the food we eat through "the food connection", the air we breathe affects our health through "the breath connection", the social and economic stresses of our inter-connected world may impact on our mental health though "the mind connection" and our close friends, family and community have a profound impact on our health through "the living connection". So it would be reasonable to assume the health and sustainability of the global environment should play a vital part in the health and well being of every individual.

Climate change, population growth, and skyrocketing meat consumption is making water scarce for two-thirds of the world's population.
Almost 4 billion people—two-thirds of the world's population—face severe water scarcity at least one month a year, according to new analysis.[36] That is far worse than previous estimates of 2 billion to 3 billion people. About 500 million struggle with this acute water shortage all year long.

Earlier estimates focused on assessing year-round water supply. That did not account for fluctuating supplies during wet and dry months and the severe water shortages that typically occur during specific times of the year, say researchers at the University of Twente in the Netherlands. The affected population lives not just in vulnerable developing countries in Asia and Africa but also in Australia, the United Kingdom, and the American West.

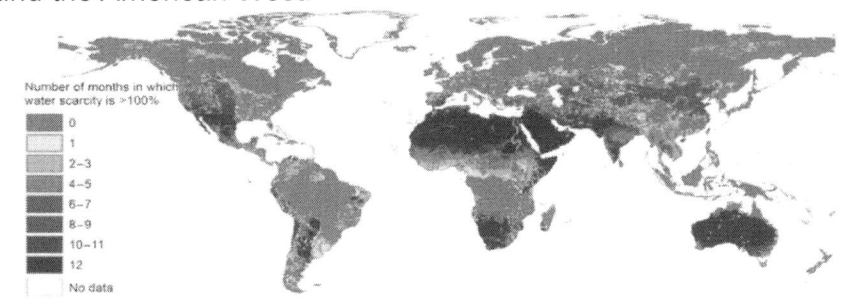

Nutrient Pollution and Coastal Dead Zones

A US National Academy of Science report[1] designates nitrogen and phosphorous pollution as the main threat to US Coastal Waters. Moreover, according to a recent EPA report 55% of all US streams are now unsuitable for aquatic life primarily due to excess nutrients.[2] The basic problem is that fertilizer runoff from corn production used primarily to feed livestock[3] and leaching from large manure ponds found at Concentrated Agricultures Feeding Operations (CAFOs), better known as factory farms, enters local streams that eventually empty into the coastal environment. Adding nutrients stimulates excess growth of phytoplankton (algae) that subsequently then die and sink to become available for bacteria to decompose in bottoms waters. As bacteria decompose the dead phytoplankton they also consume oxygen. Consequently, increasing nutrient additions indirectly leads to increases oxygen consumption by the bacteria until most or even all of the oxygen is removed from the water. With little or no oxygen in the water there can be no fish, no shrimp no marine mammals no marine life of any sort that needs oxygen to live. These regions of little or no oxygen are referred to as dead zones. The spatial extent of the Gulf of Mexico dead zone has steadily grown larger over the past several decades with the largest dead zone ever observed occurring in 2012.[4] This is not just a United States problem. Dead zones are increasing in number and size worldwide.[5] The increase in dead zones is due to the dramatic increase in worldwide use of nitrogen fertilizer to grow ever more corn for livestock feed and for ethanol production. According to personal comments made by Professor R Howarth at Cornell University, we have put more nitrogen fertilizer on the ground in the past 15 years than all the fertilizer we have used since it was invented 100 years ago!

Overfishing and Bycatch

Over the past several decades the business of commercial fishing has been transformed from familiar family-run operations to industrial fishing operations employing immense factory ships that are owned by large corporate holding companies that have little concern for conservation. The result has been a 90% decline in the abundance of valuable top-predator fish species.[6] Moreover, 82% of all major world fisheries are now either fully exploited, over exploited or in recovery according to a 2010 United Nations Food and Agriculture Organization (FAO) report.[7]

There is also moral issue to consider with regard to overfishing. Industrial-scale fishing activities take away a basic food source for poor nations with coastal communities that have only small-scale fishing capabilities that cannot compensate for the greatly reduced fish abundances created by the industrial-scale fishing operations that are supported by developed nations. Fishing efforts also cause great environmental damage due to the accidental capture of non-target species – or bycatch. The extent of the problem is a function of the global scale of a fishing operations and the type of fishing methods employed. In the case of bottom trawling for shrimp both the global scale and the methods employed lead to extremely horrific consequences.[9] [10] [11] Bottom trawling is arguably the most destructive fishing methods in terms of bycatch, but long line[12] [13] fishing & the use of fish aggregating devices (FADS)[14] come with their own highly significant bycatch problems.

Greenhouse Gas Emissions

There is a fair amount of controversy surrounding livestock's contribution to total annual greenhouse gas (GHG) emissions. An FAO report published in 2006 titled Livestock's Long Shadow: Environmental Issues and Options [17] is generally a starting point for most discussions of livestock's contributions to total GHG emissions. The FAO report estimates that livestock contributes 18% to total annual GHG emission. However, concerns have been raised about the GHG emission accounting methods used in the FAO report and about the independence of some of the authors of the FAO report that have affiliations with livestock groups. Other groups have taken a broader accounting of GHG emissions that include contributions from land changes needed for livestock development, and this accounting approach places the overall contribution by livestock at 51%.[18] Robert Goodland provides a nice discussion in a New York Times article[19] of the back and forth on the issue of livestock contributes to GHG emissions and what many feel is FAO's lowball estimate on livestock's contribution GHG emissions. For a quantitative look at the issue see the article by Tara Garnett.[20]

Soil Loss

According to the World Wildlife Fund report[21] half of all the topsoil on earth has been lost over the past 150 years. Time Magazine has a nice article on the topic of soil loss globally, and it is not very encouraging.[22] According to the article, we have about 60 years of useful topsoil left if we keep doing business as usual. The loss of soil is driven by many factors, but overgrazing by live-stock is an important one.

Feeding a Growing Human Population

Global food security in the future faces the combined forces of a rapidly growing human population and global climate change that is predicted to decrease crop yields.[23] [24] [25] The issue here is that as the planet warms and temperatures exceed the heat tolerance of major crops, yields of these crops will decline.

One way to reduce the food security problem is to shift global diets toward one that is more plant-based. For every 100 calories of grain we feed animals, we get only about 40 new calories of milk, 22 calories of eggs, 12 of chicken, 10 of pork, or 3 of beef.[26] [27] Most studies present an array of actions that are needed to address the looming food security issue, but in almost all cases one element of this array of actions is a shift to reduce global meat consumption. [28] [29] [30]

The Bigger Picture of Environmental Degradation

The full sweep of problems is described in the United Nations Environmental Program (UNEP) Millennial Ecosystem Assessment Report.[31] The report chronicles in detail the past 50 years of ecosystem degradation and describes the challenges ahead. Some of the summary points listed in the report are:

"Humans have made unprecedented changes to ecosystems in recent decades to meet growing demands for food, fresh water, fiber, and energy. These changes have helped to improve the lives of billions, but at the same time they weakened nature's ability to deliver other key services such as purification of air and water, protection from disasters, and the provision of medicines. Among the outstanding problems identified by this assessment are the dire state of many of the world's fish stocks; the intense vulnerability of the 2 billion people living in dry regions to the loss of ecosystem services, including water supply; and the growing threat to ecosystems from climate change and nutrient pollution. Human activities have taken the planet to the edge of a massive wave of species extinctions, further threatening our own well-being. The pressures on ecosystems will increase globally in coming decades unless human attitudes and actions change."

Where Do We Go From Here?

A global shift towards a vegan diet is vital to save the world from hunger, fuel poverty and the worst impacts of climate change, a UN report says. As the global population surges towards a predicted 9.1 billion people by 2050, western tastes for diets rich in meat and dairy products are unsustainable, says the report from United Nations Environment Programme's (UNEP) international panel of sustainable resource management. It says: "Impacts from agriculture are expected to increase substantially due to population growth increasing consumption of animal products. Unlike fossil fuels, it is difficult to look for alternatives: people have to eat. A substantial reduction of impacts would only be possible with a substantial worldwide diet change, Professor Edgar Hertwich, the lead author of the report, said: "Animal products cause more damage than [producing] construction minerals such as sand or cement, plastics or metals. Biomass and crops for animals are as damaging as [burning] fossil fuels."from animal product." "For example, the average water footprint per calorie for beef is 20 times larger than for cereals and starchy roots," he said. "The meat consumption per person in the world is still increasing, so the water demand grows quickly because of that." As temperatures rise because of climate change, dry places are getting drier. And burgeoning demand and more intense and longer droughts are depleting groundwater reserves. Hoekstra said 500 million people live in such regions, where water consumption is double available supplies. Vulnerable populations include 180 million people in India, 73 million in Pakistan, 27 million in Egypt, 20 million in Mexico, 20 million in Saudi Arabia, and 18 million in Yemen.

It is possible to move away from the long-held belief that humans are separate and distinct from the natural world, and to begin to think of ourselves as just one branch of nature's interconnected web of life.

Dr. Raskin calls it a need for a "Copernicus Transformation".
Back in the time of Copernicus, most would have thought it impossible if you said that you were going to convince everyone that the Earth revolved around the Sun, rather than the other way around, but it did eventually happen! So the idea of convincing everyone that they are not separate from nature & humans are not the center of the universe, but rather just one part of nature's web does not seem too far-fetched either.
We must understand that we are all connected together and to the whole dynamic, complex, living entity we call earth.

References & Resources

Ref.A1 The China Study by Dr. T Colin Canpbell & T M Campbell ISBN 978-193210066-2 p369 R.1,35

Ref.A2 The Starch Solution by Dr. J McDougall ISBN 978-1-60961-393-8, The China Study p392 R.50,72

Ref.A3 Download PDF <http://www.thebreathconnection.com/images/CardiacTBC.pdf>

Ref.A4 If Ost. A <www.thebodyconnection.co.uk>, if Rheum. arthritis The China Study p390 Refs.1 to 26

Ref.A5 The China Study p.183-201, p387 Refs.1 to 71

Ref.B1 The China study p 385 Refs. 66 to 91

Ref.B2 The China Study p 382 Refs. 1 to 58

Ref.C1 The China Study p 377 Refs.1 to 51

Ref C2 The China Study p 391 Refs. 39 to 47

Ref D1 The China Study p 381 Refs. 1 to 23

Ref D2 Visit <http://www.thefoodconnection.org.uk/diverticulosis.html>

Ref E1. Visit <http://www.thefoodconnection.org.uk/Environmental.html>

Ref F1. Visit <http://www.thefoodconnection.org.uk/Famine%20&%20malnutrition.html>

Ref G1. Visit <http://www.thefoodconnection.org.uk/gallbladder.html>

Ref G2. Visit <http://www.thefoodconnection.org.uk/Global%20warming.html>

Ref H1. Visit <http://www.thebreathconnection.com/infocard.htm>

Ref K1. The China Study p 391 Refs. 28 to 38

Ref L1. The China Study p 371 Refs.Chap 3 1,55
& visit <http://www.thefoodconnection.org.uk/Liver.html>

Ref L2. Visit <http://www.thefoodconnection.org.uk/Lupus.html>

Ref M1. The China Study p 388 Refs, 39 to 71

Ref O1. The China Study p390 Refs. 1 to 27

Ref P1. The China Study p386 Refs.93 to 102

Ref R1. Visit <http://www.thefoodconnection.org.uk/Rheumatoid.html>

Ref S1 The China Study p 377 Refs. 1 to 10 & visit <http://www.thebreathconnection.com/infocard.htm>

References & Resources

Breathing
Every Breath You Take	Paul Ameisen	0-186436728-8
Breathing Free	Teresa Hale	0-340-79496-8
Hyperventilation Syndrome	Dinah Bradley	1-85626-295-2
The Carbon Dioxide Syndrome	Jennifer & Russell Stark	978-0-473096-10-6
The Breath Connection	Michael Lingard	978-1-326-16420-1
The Buteyko Guide to Better Asthma Management	Michael Lingard	978-1-4476-4539-9

Environment
The Great Transition	Lester R Brown	978-0-393-35055-5
Climate Change	HRH Prince of Wales	978-0-718-18585-5

Health & Healing
The Stress of Life	Selye	0-07-056212-1
Not All In THe Mind	Richard Mackarness	0-330-24592-9
Measuring Health	Ann Bowling	0-335-19754-x
Natural Grace	Matthew Fox & Rupert Sheldrake	0-385-48356-2
Styes & Wedding Rings	W S Inman	0-443-01010-2
Science Synthesis & Sanity	G Scott Williamson	0-7073-0259-5
Being Me and Also Us	Alison Stallibrass	0-7073-0599-3
Love, Medicine and Miracles	Bernie Siegel	0-7126-7046-7
Why Zebras Don't Get Ulcers	Sapolsky	0-7167-3210-6
Frontiers of Health	Christine Page	0-85207-340-2
The Science & Art of Healing	Raph Twentyman	0-86315-095-0
Medicine for the Whole Person	Geoffrey Douch	0-86315-362-3
Recognising Health	Kenneth Barlow	0-9513171-0-5
Wholeness and Holiness	I D Trotter	0-9545730-0-5
Your Jaws of Life	David C Page	0-9717368-1-2
Income Inequality & Health	Ichiro Kawachi	1-56584-571-4
Nature Cure	Henry Lindlahr	1-59224-070-4
The Polarity Process	Franklyn Sills	1-85230-052-3
Medicine for the Whole Person Mythology & Spirituality	Ralph Twentyman	1-85584-182-7
Natures Alchemist	Anna Parkinson	978-0-7112-2767-5
The Caring Physician	F W Peabody	978-067409-7384
The Brains's Way of Healing	Dr. Norman Doidge	978-1-846-14424-0

Nutrition
Program Reversing Heart Disease	Dr. Dean Cornish	0-394-57565-2
Milk - The Deadly Poison	Robert Cohen	0-9659196-0-9
How Not To Die	Dr. Michael Greger	978-1-4472-8244-0
Disease Proof	David L Katz	978-1-59463-124-5
The China Study	Dr. T Colin Campbell	978-193210066-2
The Starch Solution	Dr. John McDougall	978-1-62336-027-6

References & Resources

Philosophy

Life Lessons	Elizabeth Kubler-Ross	0-7432-0811-0
Return to Nature	Alkdolf Just	0-7873-0485-9
The Connectivity Hypothesis	Ernst Laslow	0-7914-5786-9
How to Know Higher Worlds	Rudolph Steiner	0-88010-372-8
The Field of Form	Lawrence Edwards	0-903540-50-9
The Biology of Belief	Bruce H Lipton	0-9759914-7-7
The Living Energy Universe	Gary Schwartz	1-57174-455-x
A New Renaissance	David Loriman	978-086315-759-2
The Systems View of Life	Frijof Capra	978-1-107-01136-6
The Science Delusion	Rupert Sheldrake	978-1-444-72792-0
Made for Goodness	Desmond Tutu	978-1-84604-252-2
Science & the Akashic Field	Ervin Laszlo	978-159477042-5
Science of Reenchantment of the Cosmos	Ervin Laszlo	978-159477102-2
Quantum Shift in the Global Brain	Ervin Laszlo	978-159477233-7
Morphic Resonance	Rupert SheldrakeSheldrake	978-159477317-4
Whole	T Colin Campbell Philosophy	978-193785624-3

Psychology

The Luscher Colour Test	Max Luscher	0-224-61883-0
Neurophysiology	Edward Arnold	0-340-50634-2
Wisdom Intelligence & Creativity Synthesis	Steinberg	0-521-80238-5
Use Your Head	Tony Buzan	0-563-37103-x
Six Thinking Hats	De Bono	0-670-81314-1
Spiritual Intelligence	Brian Draper	978-0-7459-5321-2
The Pleasure Trap	Douglas J Lisle	978-1-57067-197-5

Environment

1. http://www8.nationalacademies.org/onpinews/newsitem.aspx?RecordID=9812
2. http://usnews.nbcnews.com/_news/2013/03/26/17475544-epa-more-than-half-of-us-rivers-unsuitable-for-aquatic-life?lite
3. http://www.nationalgeographic.com/foodfeatures/feeding-9-billion/
4. http://science.time.com/2013/06/19/this-years-gulf-of-mexico-dead-zone-could-be-the-biggest-on-record/Diaz, R. J. and R Rosenberg (2008) Spreading dead zones and consequences for marine ecosystems. Science 321 (5891): 926-929 Myers and Worm (2003). Rapid worldwide depletion of predatory fish communities. Nature 423: 280-283
5. http://www.fao.org/docrep/013/i1820e/i1820e.pdf
6. http://ngm.nationalgeographic.com/2007/04/global-fisheries-crisis/fisheries-crisis-interactive
7. http://oceana.org/sites/default/files/reports/Trawling_BZ_10may10_toAudrey.pdf
8. http://www.amnh.org/explore/science-bulletins/bio/documentaries/will-the-fish-return/trawling-takes-a-toll

References & Resources

Environment continued

11. http://www.fao.org/docrep/w6602e/w6602e09.htm
12. Gallagher, A.J. et. al. (2014). Vulnerability of oceanic sharks as pelagic longline bycatch. Global Ecology and Conservation 1:50-59
13. http://www.audubon.org/magazine/september-october-2013/will-world-adopt-sustainable-longline
14. http://www.pewtrusts.org/en/multimedia/data-visualizations/2013/proliferating-use-of-fish-aggregating-de
15. Naylor, R. L. et al. (2009) Feeding aquaculture in an era of finite resources. PNAS 106(42):15103-15110
16. Pikitch, E.K. et al. (2014) The global contribution of forage fish to marine fisheries and ecosystems. Fish and Fisheries 15(1):43-64
17. http://www.fao.org/docrep/010/a0701e/a0701e00.HTM
18. http://www.worldwatch.org/node/6294
19. http://bittman.blogs.nytimes.com/2012/07/11/fao-yields-to-meat-industry-pressure-on-climate-change/
20. Garnett, T. (2011) Where are the best opportunities for reducing greenhouse gas emissions in the food system (including the food chain) Food Policy, 36:S23-S32
21. https://www.worldwildlife.org/threats/soil-erosion-and-degradation
22. http://world.time.com/2012/12/14/what-if-the-worlds-soil-runs-out/
23. Battisti, D.S. and R. L. Naylor (2009) Historical warnings of future food insecurity with unprecedented seasonal heat. Science 323(5911): 240-244
24. Wheeler, T. and J. von Braun (2013) Climate Change Impacts on Global Food Security. Science 341 (6145):508-513
25. Food & Agriculture Organization (FAO). How to Feed the World in 2050.
26. http://www.nationalgeographic.com/foodfeatures/feeding-9-billion/
27. http://www.cam.ac.uk/research/news/changing-global-diets-is-vital-to-reducing-climate-change
28. http://news.yahoo.com/blogs/the-lookout/vegetarian-2050-190426669.html
29. http://www.huffingtonpost.ca/2012/08/27/vegetarian-diet-scientist_n_1834182.html
30. http://www.theguardian.com/global-development/2012/aug/26/food-shortages-world-vegetarianism
31. http://www.unep.org/maweb/en/Reports.aspx
32. http://www.geo.cornell.edu/ocean/1_Homework_Assignment_fall_2014.pdf
33. http://www.health.gov/dietaryguidelines/2015-scientific-report/ (See chapters 4 and 5 of the report or read the Executive Summary http://www.health.gov/dietaryguidelines/2015-scientific-report/02-executive-summary.asp
34. http://www.health.gov/dietaryguidelines/dga2015/comments/
35. https://www.youtube.com/watch?v=FS7o4g5kzMM
36. https://youtu.be/XDdWiY6xje0

Index

A Story about Pan Killers & The Red Flashing Light 19
Abdomen 12
Adrenals 10
Allergies 29, 51, 58
Allergies, Sinusitis & Hayfever 58
Alzheimer's Disease & Dementia   29
Andrew Taylor Still 22
Angina   30
Anus   12
Anxiety & Panic Attacks   62
Appendix 12
Arthritis   30
Asthma   56
At Peckham   86
Auto-immune Diseases   30
B12 Supplements   47
Babies   14
Babies and how you can help 16
Beta-agonist Reliever Medications   56
Better Health & A Long Active Life   28
Bladder   11
Bone fractures   43
Boosting your child's immune system   16
Bowel Cancer   31
Breast Cancer   32
Can I exercise my mechanical problems away? 20,33
Capnography   65, 68
Carbon dioxide   51
Cateracts & Macular Degeneration   35,36
Check Your Own Breathing   65
Children's Stuctural Problems 14
Circulation   32
Control Pause   65
Copernicus Transformation   94
Coronary Heart Disease   33,34,35
Counselling   70
CPAP Machines   60
Dental & Orthodontic Problems   63
Diabetes 36,37
Diaphragm   9
Dietary Q & A's (Destroying old myths on diet) 46, 47
Diverticulitis   38
Diverticulosis   38
Do you have any of these symptoms?   52
Doctors Comments Worldwide 66
Does it really matter what I eat?   24
Dr. Caldwell B. Esselstyn, Jr   35
Dr. Callaghan's Thought Field Therapy 73
Dr. G. Scott Williamson   77

99

Dr. Glen Domam   70
Dr. Innes Pearse   77
Dr. John Flutter   63
Dr. John McDougall 39
Dr. Richard Mackarness   29
Dr. Roy Swank   42
Dr. T Colin Campbell & Thomas M Campbell   31
Dr. W G Robertson 40
Duodenum   10
Ear problems   9
Earache relief   16
Early age of first menstruation 32
Eczema 57
EMDR - Eye Movement Desensitisation 74
Emotional Freedom Technique or EFT   70, 73
Emphysema and COPD   57
Environment Destruction & Our Diet   38, 91, 93
Ethology & Pathology   88
Facial pains   9
Famine & Malnutrition   38, 92
Feeding a Growing Human Population   92
Feet   12
Finance 87
Fundamental Concepts of Body Mechanics   4
Further Work Based on First Findings   81
Gall Bladder   11
Gall Bladder Problems   39
General Health, Fitness Sport & Wellbeing   62
Getting to Know Your Body   6
Global Warming & Our Diet   39, 40, 92
Glue Ear 15
Good Body Mechanics are the Basis of Good Health.   3
Greenhouse Gas Emissions   92
Heart   11
High blood cholesterol   32
High Blood Pressure   33, 51, 61
High levels of female hormones   32,33
Holism or Wholism 70
How can my back pain be connected to my heart problem? 6
How do I know I need physical therapy? 19
How do you choose a physical therapist?   21
How's Your Body Knowledge?   3
Hypertension   40
Hyperventilation   65
Hypnotherapy   70, 72
Insulin-like Growth Factor 1, IGF-1   44,45
Is your knee problem really a knee problem?   16
Is your neck problem really a neck problem?   17
Kidney Stones   40, 41
Kidneys 10
Knee   12
Lao-Tzu (circa 4th century BC).   50
Large Intestine   10

Late menopause   32
Leonardo da Vinci   70
Life Coaching   75
Liver   11
Liver Cancer   41
Lower limbs   12
Lungs   10
Lupus   42
Lymph Circulation   11
Mind Myths & Facts 76
Mindfulness   70
More Information on Whole Plant Diet   48
Multiple Sclerosis   42, 43
Neck pains   8
Neuro Linguistic Programming NLP   70, 71
Nijmegen Questionnaire   65
Normal Breathing   50
Nutrient Pollution and Coastal Dead Zones   90
Oesophagus   11
Orthodontics   15
Osteoporosis   43
Overfishing and Bycatch   91
Overweeight, Obesity   33
Pancreas 10
Patient Testimonials 67
Pioneer Health Centre   77
Posture   13
Professor Konstantin Buteyko 49, 53
Prostate   12
Prostate Cancer   44
Refernce books on Whole Plant Diet   48
Rheumatoid Arthritis   45
Sanity   88
Sciatic Nerve   12
Sexual Organs   12
Sleep Apnoea   60
Small intestine   11
Smoking   33
Snoring   59
Soil Loss   92
Spleen   10
Start by checking your own diet   25
Statins   33
Stomach   11
Stress   33,49
Stress & The Breath Connection   54
Stroke   45
The 4LeafSurvey   25,26
The Bigger Picture of Environmental Degradation   93
The Body Heals Itself if Conditions are Right   4, 5
The Bohr Effect   51, 60
The Breath Connection & Technology   68
The Breath Connection Training Course 64

The Breath Connection Training Courses   55
The Building Again 83
The Buteyko Method & Clinical Trials   55, 56
The Calgary Trial Canada 2007   55
The China Study   31, 32, 34, 37, 40, 41, 42, 43, 44
The Demise of Physical Therapy (Osteopathy in Particular) 22
The Environment Connection 89
The Experiment   79
The Eyes 8
The First Conclusions   80
The Food Connection   23
The Framlingham Study   45
The Fundamental Concepts of Body Mechanics   4
The Gisborne Trial New Zealand 2003   55
The Head 8
The Hidden Workings of Your Spine Revealed   7
The Living Connection   77
The Mater Hospital Trial Brisbane 1998 55
The Peckham Experiment   77
The People Again   84
The Plastic Brain   69
The Plastic Brain - How can we change it?   70
The Rise of Reductionism & the Fall of Wholism   5
The Venturi Effect   59
Thyroid & Heart   9
Upper limbs   10
Uterus   11
Vitamin D 44
Vocal chords   9
Weight Problems   46
What Controls our Breathing? 51
What is Health?   78
What is Your Health Risk with Your Present Diet?   27
Where Do We Go From Here? 93
Why is CO2 so important?   51
Why is Hyperventilation not Easily Noticed ?   53
You are what you eat!   24
Young Children   16